Secrets of Success: Getting into Specialty Training

Edited by

Philip J Smith BMedSci(Hons) BMBS MRCP(London)
ST4 in Academic Clinical Fellow in Gastroenterology, London
Deanery, London, UK

Manoj Ramachandran BSc(Hons) MBBS(Hons) MRCS(Eng)
FRSC(Tr&Orth)
Consultant Trauma and Orthopaedic Surgeon, Barts and The
London NHS Trust, London, UK; Honorary Senior Lecturer, William
Harvey Research Institute, Barts and The London School of Medicine
& Dentistry, London, UK

Marc A Gladman MBBS PhD MRCOG MRCS(Eng) FRCS(Gen
Surg)
UKCRC Clinical Lecturer in Surgery, Centre for Academic Surgery,
Institute of Cell & Molecular Science, Barts and The London School
of Medicine & Dentistry, London, UK

Associate Editor

Elizabeth A Owen MBBS BMedSci(Hons) MRCPCH
ST3 in Paediatrics, London Deanery, London, UK

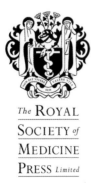

The ROYAL
SOCIETY of
MEDICINE
PRESS Limited

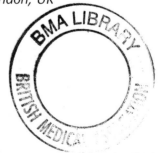

Published by the Royal Society of Medicine Press Ltd
1 Wimpole Street, London W1G 0AE, UK
Tel: +44 (0)20 7290 2921
Fax: +44 (0)20 7290 2929
E-mail: publishing@rsmpress.co.uk

British Library Cataloguing in Publication Data.
A catalogue record for this book is available from the British Library

ISBN: 978-1-85315-893-3

Distribution in Europe and Rest of the World:
Marston Book Services Ltd
PO Box 269
Abingdon
Oxon OX14 4YN, UK
Tel: +44 (0)1235 465500
Fax: +44 (0)1235 465555
Email: direct.order@marston.co.uk

Distribution in USA and Canada:
Royal Society of Medicine Press Ltd
c/o BookMasters Inc
30 Amberwood Parkway
Ashland, OH 44805, USA
Tel: +1 800 247 6553/ +1 800 266 5564
Fax: +1 410 281 6883
Email: order@bookmasters.com

Distribution in Australia and New Zealand:
Elsevier Australia
30–52 Smidmore Street
Marrickville NSW 2204, Australia
Tel: +61 2 9517 8999
Fax: +61 2 9517 2249
Email: service@elsevier.com.au

Typeset by IMH(Cartrif), EH20 9DX, Scotland, UK
Printed in the UK by Bell & Bain, Glasgow, UK

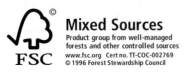

Mixed Sources
Product group from well-managed
forests and other controlled sources
www.fsc.org Cert no. TT-COC-002769
© 1996 Forest Stewardship Council

Contents

Contributors

Philip J Smith BMedSci(Hons) BMBS MRCP(London)
ST4 in Academic Clinical Fellow in Gastroenterology, London
Deanery, London, UK

Manoj Ramachandran BSc(Hons) MBBS(Hons) MRCS(Eng)
FRCS (Tr&Orth)
Consultant Trauma and Orthopaedic Surgeon, Barts and The
London NHS Trust, London, UK; Honorary Senior Lecturer,
William Harvey Research Institute, Barts and The London
School of Medicine & Dentistry, London, UK

Marc A Gladman MBBS PhD MRCOG MRCS(Eng)
FRCS(Gen Surg)
UKCRC Clinical Lecturer in Surgery, Centre for Academic
Surgery, Institute of Cell & Molecular Science, Barts and The
London School of Medicine & Dentistry, London, UK

Elizabeth A Owen MBBS BMedSci(Hons) MRCPCH
ST3 in Paediatrics, London Deanery, London, UK

Zohra Ali MBBS(Hons) BSc(Hons) MRCP(London)
ST3 in Medical Oncology, Yorkshire and the Humber Deanery,
Leeds, UK

Beverley Almeida BMedSci(Hons) BMBS MRCPCH
ST4 in Paediatrics, London Deanery, London, UK

Anna Barrow MBBS BA(Oxon)
CT1 ACCS (Anaesthetics), London Deanery, London, UK

Megan Crofts MBChB
CT2 Core Medical Trainee, London Deanery, London, UK

Jasdeep K Gill MBChB(Hons)
ST1 in General Practice, London Deanery, London, UK

Chris Godeseth BMedSci(Hons) BMBS MRCS(Ed)
Formerly ST2 in Trauma and Orthopaedics, East Midlands
Deanery, Nottingham and Leicester, UK

Shalini Kawar MBBS BSc DRCOG DFSRH
ST3 in General Practice, London Deanery, London, UK

Kamaldeep Kaur Manak MBBS BMedSci
ST2 in General Practice, London Deanery, London, UK

David Middleton BMedSci(Hons) BMBS MRCPsych
ST4 in Psychiatry, East of England Deanery, Cambridge, UK

Luke Moore MBChB MRCP(London) DTM&H
ST4 in Infectious Diseases and Microbiology, London Deanery,
London, UK

Rachel Nicholson MB BChir MRCS
ST2 in Obstetrics and Gynaecology, West Midlands Deanery,
Birmingham,UK

Sukhjinder Nijjer MBChB(Hons) BSc(Hons) MRCP(London)
ST4 in Cardiology, London Deanery, London, UK

Shilpa Patel MBBS BSc(Hons) MRCP(London)
ST3 in Radiology, London Deanery, London, UK

Mark J Portou MB ChB(Hons) MRCS(Eng)
ST3 in General Surgery, London Deanery, London, UK

Anne Swift MBChB(Hons)
ST2 in Public Health, East of England Deanery, Cambridge, UK

Jane Walker BSc MBBS
ST3 in Histopathology, West Midlands Deanery, Birmingham,
UK

The philosophy of 'Maximize *Your* Medical Career'

It is now over 16 years since we first met at medical school, united by a passion for education and a desire to excel in our medical careers. During this time we have been working together and have actively designed and delivered numerous products to facilitate the development of medical students and junior doctors. To this day, we are surprised by the lack of formal career guidance and development available for doctors. Professional development for doctors is complex, involving the acquisition of numerous clinical and non-clinical skills. Some individuals are fortunate enough to encounter altruistic peers or senior colleagues who act as mentors, providing informal instruction based on their own experiences. Frequently, however, it is a process of chance or self-tuition for the majority of doctors, some of whom never acquire the necessary skills, particularly non-clinical attributes (e.g. succeeding in job applications, leadership, motivation, teamworking).

The concept of 'Maximize YOUR Medical Career' has been developed by us to specifically address the void in the development of medical students and junior doctors. Our aim is to provide mentorship, comprehensive guidance and professional development for individual doctors to facilitate career progression through a portfolio of innovative products that reflect our enthusiasm, energy and unique style. We hope that you and your future careers can benefit from the knowledge of our own experiences. All too often, we are told to aim to achieve 'competence' in medicine. Our philosophy is to never be satisfied with settling for this, but instead we urge you to strive for 'excellence' and being the best that you can possibly be!

The 'Secrets of Success' series of books embodies this philosophy. This third instalment is aimed at helping you secure a job in your chosen specialty.

Marc A Gladman and Manoj Ramachandran

Preface

'The life so short, the craft so long to learn'

Hippocrates on medicine

With the advent of Modernising Medical Careers and the formation of specialty training, junior doctors now have a streamlined structure from which they can graduate to become the consultants of tomorrow. This is the final endpoint after many years of hard work and dedication, which, in some cases, started over two decades before at medical school. Reaching consultant level may well be the fulfilment of a dream – reaching the pinnacle of your chosen vocation in your chosen specialty.

It is not always easy to make the right choices for yourself when the world of medicine offers so much diversity. Indeed, specialty training is now a very significant crossroad in a junior doctor's career – choosing the most appropriate direction can be mind-boggling. You need to be realistic, and have clear goals and objectives to succeed in specialty training – often recognizing these before setting out on the first few premature steps into a field. It is also crucial not to lose sight of what is really important to you as a person – is it the job you do, the specialty, or the location you do it in? If all of these are equally important then although this is an entirely reasonable goal, you need to ensure you are at the top of your game, so that you can achieve all that you want.

This book aims to guide applicants for specialty training posts through the various stresses and challenges of the application and interview processes to enable candidates to increase their own chances of successfully securing their dream job. The book is divided into five sections, each of which may be used in isolation or in conjunction with the others. It aims to guide and assist rather than give verbatim answers to both generic and specialty-specific questions, so that readers can mould their own answers using a number of approaches to different questions. As the book's title 'Secrets of Success' suggests, its credibility is based upon the fact it is written for specialty trainees by specialty trainees from a wide range of specialties – all of whom can provide a real-life insight into the best way to get into a chosen specialty. All the contributors have worked extremely hard to ensure that the information within this book is relevant and as up to date as possible, so as to best support future cohorts of trainees, although undoubtedly some people may have differing opinions on how to approach the specialty training recruitment process.

It must be stressed that the aim of this book is not to provide a set of 'perfect' responses to every possible question that might be encountered in the specialty training applications and interviews. Rather, it aims to teach you certain skills that will provide you with the necessary tools, so that you may successfully complete your own application when the time comes. *Allied to this point, we must urge you not be tempted to copy or modify any of the examples included in this book when completing your own application.* Not only is plagiarism a serious offence, but you will have completely missed the point of this book if you intend to use it for that purpose. Further, you will face serious consequences if caught – *you have been warned!*

Good luck!

PJS, MR, MAG

Acknowledgements

To Beverley, Mum, Dad and all my family – I love you all, thank you for your constant love and support in everything I do.

PJS

We are grateful to the contributors for all their hard work, produced in a timely fashion.

We should like to offer our most sincere thanks to everyone at RSM Press Ltd who has supported this project (and for their patience in allowing its completion!), particularly Sarah Ogden, Sarah McConalogue and Peter Richardson.

PJS, MG, MAR

Key to icons

 Top Tip

 Question

 Facts and Figures

Danger

Ask the Expert

Homework

SECTION A
Applying for specialty training

1 Introduction to specialty training

Mark J Portou

'Modernising Medical Careers'

Postgraduate medical education in the UK underwent radical reform on 1 August 2005 with the implementation of the first phase of the Government initiative 'Modernising Medical Careers' (MMC).

Unfinished business: the genesis of MMC

Problems with the Senior House Officer (SHO) grade were highlighted in the 2002 report by the Chief Medical Officer of England: *Unfinished Business: Proposals for Reform of the Senior House Officer Grade*. The earliest principles of MMC were first conceived in this document. This report identified that half of the SHO jobs were short-term 'stand-alone' posts with no association with training rotations. Five key principles for SHO reform were suggested, and stated that training should:

- be programme-based
- be broadly-based, to begin with, for all trainees
- provide individually tailored programmes to meet specific needs
- be time-capped
- support movement of doctors into and out of training and between training programmes.

In addition, the use of a standardized curriculum was suggested. Robust and consistent assessment tools would be implemented, and the selection process was to be overhauled, by creating a national centralized application procedure.

The structure of MMC

On exiting medical school, the newly qualified doctor will enter a 2-year Foundation Programme. Full registration with the General Medical Council (GMC) is applied for following successful completion of year 1 of the Foundation Programme (F1). Foundation year 2 (F2), is a continuation of 'generic' training started in F1. It was intended that F2 would provide the trainee with the opportunity to experience specialties not previously available to juniors, such as microbiology, biochemistry, histopathology, public health and psychiatry.

After successful completion of the Foundation Programme, the doctor then progresses to specialty training (ST) via competitive entry. ST programmes include all hospital disciplines such as medicine, surgery, anaesthetics, paediatrics and psychiatry, with general practice having a different application process.

The initial intention was that these ST programmes would run seamlessly from entry until attainment of a senior medical appointment. As recommended in *Unfinished Business*, the selection process for entry into ST programmes in 2007 was via a centralized, computer-based application system. An online Medical Training and Application Service (MTAS) was created for this purpose, although no one could have predicted the well publicized debacle that ensued. Serious doubts emerged regarding the robustness of the shortlisting process and selection of doctors for ST posts. Concerns regarding the validity of the questions and marking procedures to accurately discriminate led to the Department of Health setting up a review group comprising Royal Colleges and the British Medical Association (BMA). Subsequently, an independent enquiry was commissioned, headed by Sir John Tooke.

The Tooke report

This independent enquiry was established by the Health Secretary in April 2007 into the failure of the MTAS and the feasibility of the current state of MMC. This enquiry was far reaching and engaging, examining minutes of meetings, interviewing the key players, with online consultations and forums where juniors from across the country were able to convey their views and solutions regarding the subject to the investigating team.

An interim report was published in October 2007. The response and feedback to the interim report were impressive, and perhaps reflect to some degree an anti-MMC backlash by the profession. Of the 45 recommendations in the interim report, 87% were 'agreed' or 'strongly agreed' with. Following this period of consultation, the final report was published in January 2008. The enquiry makes 47 recommendations which, if adopted, will once again have dramatic consequences for the structure of postgraduate medical education.

Tooke report recommendations

A key recommendation of the report was to 'uncouple' the Foundation years. Tooke recommended that F1 should continue but that F2 should be incorporated into ST programmes. However, the final report acknowledges that the Foundation Programme has been a relatively successful MMC policy and thus it is unclear whether this recommendation will be implemented.

After the Foundation Programme, doctors would apply to enter 'Core Specialty Training', in one of four stems (see below), which would provide 'broad-based' training lasting for 2 or 3 years with continued emphasis on competency acquisition. Run-through training would continue, but after the first year of core training and only in certain specialties. Core training is intended to be via six 6-month placements, and will follow curricula adapted from the current ST years. In response to criticism over the inflexibility of the 'run-through' training model of MMC, it is proposed that Core Specialty Training should be general enough to allow flexibility, and allow competitive transfer between the core stems in years 1 and 2, allowing trainees to change their mind regarding career direction.

Following completion of Core Specialty Training, Tooke suggests competitive application to Higher Specialty Training, via a standard, specialty-specific application form, and using individual curricula vitae (CVs). These applications would be made several times per year, and use national selection centres to assess 'knowledge, skills and aptitudes'. Final selection, following the shortlisting process, will be via structured interviews.

Higher Specialty Training will take the trainee through to Certificate of Completion of Training (CCT). Post-training doctors are then separated into 'specialists' and 'consultants', with further college exams/training perhaps the discriminating factor.

In addition to the changes highlighted above, the Tooke report also made many other recommendations. The report recognized that doctors, particularly those in training, have an undefined role within the modern multidisciplinary teams, and thus it is currently unsuitable to use 'outcome-focused' education methods. It is advised that clarification of the role of doctors at all levels, including service contributions, requires urgent consideration. It was also recommended that a new body, the NHS: Medical Education England (NHS: MEE), should oversee postgraduate medical education in England including defining its underpinning principles and, among other responsibilities, holding training budgets.

2 Specialty training across the specialties

Philip J Smith, Manoj Ramachandran and Marc A Gladman

Introduction

The majority of applicants to specialty training (ST) will have successfully navigated their way through Foundation training, although some applicants will be overseas nationals (EU and non-EU applicants). Irrespective of the route followed, satisfactory achievement (and demonstration) of the Foundation training competencies are a prerequisite for application to ST.

The current situation

Currently, there are different training offers for different specialties, to fit the particular needs of the specialty. Some specialties continue to offer run-through training (ST1, ST2, etc.), while others are 'uncoupled' and offer a 2- or 3-year core training (CT) programme (CT1, CT2, CT3). CT is then followed by an open competition to enter higher ST at ST3 onwards (ST4 for psychiatry and emergency medicine). The terminology for CT is CT1, CT2 (and CT3 for psychiatry and emergency medicine), agreed with the Postgraduate Medical Education and Training Board (PMETB).

Offer of run-through training in 2009	Offer with uncoupling in 2009 (Core training followed by open competition to higher ST)
Obstetrics and gynaecology	General medicine
Ophthalmology	Anaesthesia
Paediatrics and child health	Clinical oncology
General practice	Psychiatry
Public health medicine	Occupational medicine
Neurosurgery	Emergency medicine
Histopathology	*Cardiothoracic surgery*
Chemical pathology	*General surgery*
Medical microbiology	*Oral maxillofacial surgery*
Clinical radiology	*Otolaryngology (ENT)*
	Paediatric surgery
	Plastic surgery
	Trauma and orthopaedic surgery
	Urology

The entry competition between CT and higher ST will be open to all eligible applicants (including those working in non-training posts or otherwise not on CT programmes). This will provide opportunities in future years to enter training at a higher level for those people who were not previously successful in securing a CT or run-through training post.

For those specialties where training is uncoupled, CT is offered to a larger pool of applicants, without the need for fixed-term specialty training appointments (FTSTAs). However, FTSTA1 and FTSTA2 will continue in run-through specialties to add to the opportunities for doctors to develop their training experience and improve their chances of entering later to ST.

A summary of Modernising Medical Careers (MMC) postgraduate training in England is shown in Figure 2.1.

Progress through specialty (and core) training is subject to the satisfactory completion of the Annual Review of Competence Progression (ARCP), with satisfactory achievement of the expected milestones set out for run-through trainees in their chosen specialty.

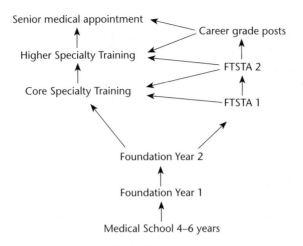

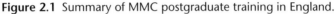

Figure 2.1 Summary of MMC postgraduate training in England.

Within the uncoupled specialties, the CT programmes are available in:

- core medical training
- core surgical training
- acute care common stem (ACCS)
- core psychiatric training.

Each of these will be discussed in more detail below.

Core training programmes

As in Foundation training, your time is divided between a number of specialties over, in most cases, a 2-year training period. Such rotations aim to provide a broad base of experience before subsequent specialization. Typically, attachments may consist of three 4-month rotations or two 6-month rotations over the course of a year.

Core medical training

In core medical training, a typical training programme may take the form of six 4-month attachments or three 4-month attachments and two 6-month attachments – these may be based in one hospital or a number of hospitals, ideally within a similar geographical area within that deanery. For example:

CT1: Elderly care medicine/oncology/acute medicine
CT2: Intensive care/cardiology/HIV medicine

Within this training programme, doctors are expected to develop a broad base of experience, as well as completing all the core competencies expected within that 2-year programme. ARCPs are held at 8, 16 and 23 months during the programme. These must be successfully completed to progress. Such assessments will be completed with your assigned educational supervisor and programme director in your training region.

After successful completion of CT1 and CT2 you can apply competitively for any ST3 post in any medical specialty.

Core surgical training

For the majority of surgical specialties, entry into run-through ST will only be possible following successful completion of a CT programme and thus will be at ST3 level. The core programme is termed 'CT in surgery in general (generic)'. In common with medicine, a typical training programme may take the form of six 4-month attachments or three 4-month attachments and two 6-month attachments and encompasses many of the surgical specialties. For example:

CT1: General surgery/trauma and orthopaedic surgery
CT2: Plastic surgery/cardiothoracic surgery/otolaryngology
      (ENT)

It should be noted, however, that at least for the 2009 application process, four deaneries (Northern, West Midlands, North Western and Yorkshire and the Humber) are offering run-through as well as CT in trauma and orthopaedic surgery. Satisfactory achievement of competencies at CT1 and CT2 (documented via ARCP assessments) and completion of the Intercollegiate Membership of the Royal College of Surgeons (MRCS) examination are prerequisites for applying for ST posts (at ST3 level) in one of the surgical specialties, i.e. cardiothoracic surgery, general surgery, otolaryngology (ENT), paediatric surgery, plastic surgery, trauma and orthopaedic surgery or urology.

Acute care common stem (ACCS)

This specialty is unique in that there are three themes, aimed at developing training for a career in acute medicine, anaesthetics and emergency medicine. Consequently, a 2-year core rotation (CT1 and CT2 ACCS) will involve time in areas such as intensive care, accident and emergency, medical admission units and operating theatres. Again, to progress into the next year, satisfactory completion of the appropriate competencies must be met.

1. *Emergency medicine themed ACCS rotation*: doctors completing this theme do a third year in emergency medicine. They may then competitively apply for entry into ST4 emergency medicine.
2. *Anaesthesia intensive care medicine themed ACCS rotation*: doctors completing this theme do a third year in anaesthesia at the CT2 level. They may then competitively apply for ST3 anaesthesia.
3. *Acute medicine themed ACCS rotation*: doctors completing this 2-year ACCS programme have adequate experience to apply for ST3 in acute medicine.

Core psychiatric training

Psychiatric training is different in that CT goes from CT1 to CT3, with an open competition to apply for an ST4 job.

Typically the rotations involve two 6-month placements each year. For example:

CT1: General adult psychiatry/old age psychiatry
CT2: Child and adolescent psychiatry/crisis resolution and home treatment
CT3: Learning disability psychiatry/general adult psychiatry

The idea is to give a broad-based experience in the CT1–CT3 years with further ST from ST4 onwards. Assessment during this time involves completion of a number of assessments including Assessment of Clinical Expertise (ACEs) and mini-ACEs, which are designed to provide feedback on skills essential to the provision of good care during a whole clinical encounter or part clinical encounter, respectively. Case-based discussions (CbD) and mini-

Peer Assessment Tool (PAT) are also used. Each year psychiatry trainees have to pass an ARCP.

These assessments are used also to enable you to sit the MRCPsych examinations – with the numbers of these assessments completed being used as a measure as to when you can sit Papers I, II, III and, finally, the Clinical Assessment of Skills and Competencies (CASC) examination.

Progression from core training to specialty training

Progressing from CT2 to ST3 in medicine, surgery and ACCS is a significant transition point and is the equivalent of promotion from the senior house officer to specialist registrar grade in the old training system. Not only does it provide the challenge of increased autonomy and responsibility, for many it finally offers the opportunity to specialize in their chosen discipline within medicine, surgery or acute care. However, this transition point represents yet another hurdle to securing the all important run-through ST post. Applicants are reminded that the competition is again fierce as core trainees, FTSTA post holders and career grade posts are eligible to apply to the uncoupled specialties. The successful appointment to a ST post and award of a National Training Number (NTN) (see below) guarantees training in this specialty through to the award of the Certificate of Completion of Training (CCT). The length of time from the point of entry into ST to CCT depends on the individual specialty.

Special considerations

Radiology is interesting in that applications are invited from F2 doctors, as well as ST1–ST3 and CT1–CT3 trainees from other specialties, as radiology trainees have traditionally had experience (and frequently passed Royal College examinations) in another specialty such as medicine or surgery, prior to entry.

Clinical academic training

It is possible to embark on an academic career as early as medical school (by completing an MB/PhD). Further opportunities are available within the Foundation Programme, with the formation of Academic Foundation year posts. With the advent of the Walport report, a more streamlined and attractive structured career pathway has been devised for doctors wishing to pursue a clinical academic career, leading to the formation of two new positions: the Academic Clinical Fellowship (ACF) and Clinical Lecturer (CL) posts (see Figure 2.2).

For doctors in the early years of training an ACF provides an excellent clinical and academic training environment to help prepare a competitive application for a training fellowship for a higher degree. Funding is available for a maximum of 3 years and during this time trainees spend 75% of their time undertaking traditional (and identical) clinical training and 25% in academic training. It is possible to apply for an ACF while holding a run-through 'clinical' training post or an FTSTA. In addition, trainees already holding a clinical NTN who are subsequently selected for an integrated academic/clinical programme will have their NTN converted to an NTN(A) or receive an NTN(A) in the appropriate specialty. Application for an ACF may be at different levels (ST1, ST2, ST3, and ST4 for Psychiatry and Paediatrics), depending on specialty and whether applicants meet the appropriate personal specifications and are eligible for entry at that level.

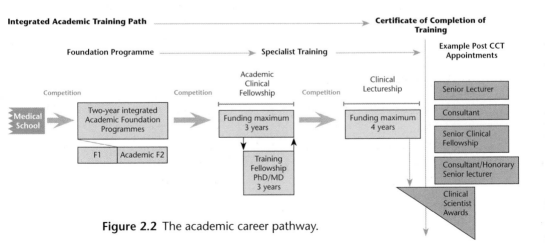

Figure 2.2 The academic career pathway.

ACFs are expected to complete a higher degree, e.g. PhD or MD(Res) and, if successful, are eligible to apply for a Clinical Lectureship post, which provides an opportunity to complete postdoctoral research or educational training while completing their ST. Funding for this is typically for a maximum of 4 years, during which time training is split equally between clinical and academic activities. Further information for those interested in pursuing an academic career can be found on the websites for the NIHR Coordinating Centre for Research Capacity Development (www.nccrcd.nhs.uk) and MMC (www.mmc.nhs.uk).

National Training Numbers (NTNs)

Securing a run-through ST post within a deanery leads to the receipt of an NTN, which trainees retain until award of the CCT. NTNs are issued following completion of 'Form R' and registration for postgraduate ST. The NTN has three purposes:

- It acts as a passport taking trainees to CCT if progress is satisfactory.
- It helps with workforce planning by helping to determine how many doctors are in training at once.
- It assists with education planning and management, as it keeps track of trainees' progress.

Top tips for progressing into specialty/core training

- Research your chosen specialty well in advance – visit the deanery and MMC websites and ask senior colleagues about working in that specialty.

- Read the 'Gold Guide' on the MMC website – it will help clarify any additional questions you have about applying into your chosen field.

- Read the personal specifications on the deanery and MMC websites to ensure that you are eligible for the specialty and level that you wish to apply for.

3 The application process and scoring

Philip J Smith

National versus local recruitment

After the Medical Training and Application Service (MTAS) debacle, one of the recommendations of the Tooke report was to revert to local, deanery-led applications for the majority of the specialties. However, some specialties are recruiting by means of a national process handled by one deanery acting on behalf of all others. These exceptions to locally organized recruitment are justified as follows.

1. Small specialties with very few posts available, when it is better for recruitment to be organized centrally. Examples include:
   - Cardiothoracic surgery at specialty training year 3 (ST3) (West Midlands)
   - Plastic surgery at ST3 (London Deanery)
   - Neurosurgery at all levels (South Yorkshire and South Humber Deanery)
   - Public health at all levels (East Midlands Deanery)
   - Histopathology at all levels (London Deanery)
   - Academic Clinical Fellowships at all levels (National Institute for Health Research Capacity Development Programme).
2. Larger specialties with standardized shortlisting and interview processes and scoring systems across the country, allowing accurate comparison between deaneries. Examples include:
   - Paediatrics and Child Health at all levels (Royal College of Paediatrics and Child Health)

- Obstetrics and gynaecology at all levels (Royal College of Obstetricians and Gynaecologists)
- General practice at all levels (National Recruitment Office for General Practice Training).

All other specialties have taken the recommendations of Tooke and are running local, deanery-led applications. Such locally-led systems have the advantage that candidates can target their applications to the areas of the country in which they wish to work/live. However, if a candidate decides to apply to lots of different deaneries this will mean completing numerous different application forms! It should also be noted that when you apply to a deanery, and are offered a place, it does not guarantee that you will work in a particular hospital; it just means you have an offer of employment within that area. Subsequently, you are then ranked according to your scoring in the interviews and this will decide which post and hospital you are assigned to. Some deaneries, particularly those that cover a large geographical area, often allow you to rank your preference of location/posts (e.g. in the London/Kent, Surrey and Sussex deanery, those selected for interview would be allowed to express a preference for north-east London, etc.).

Selection processes do vary slightly from deanery to deanery, although the overall principles remain approximately the same. Most deaneries will run an application process from early January, which will be available and advertised on each deanery's website as well as on the Modernising Medical Careers (MMC) website (www.mmc.nhs.uk) and on the BMJ careers website (www.bmjcareers.co.uk). For those applicants who are unsuccessful, a second round is available where the remaining ST positions will be filled.

Once you have accepted a job, you MUST withdraw from any further applications, interviews or offers. Deaneries state that the offer is made on the condition that you have not accepted other offers and that you withdraw from other applications. If it is discovered that you have accepted an offer after already accepting another post, that offer will be withdrawn and you will be reported to the General Medical Council (GMC). There are, however, some exceptions to this rule.

- If you have accepted a fixed-term specialty training appointment (FTSTA), you may continue to compete for a run-through training post or for uncoupled training programmes that are offering 2 years or more of core training (CT). However, you may not apply for another post that only offers 1 year of training.
- If you have accepted a run-through training post, you are eligible to apply for an Academic Clinical Fellowship post.
- If you are already in a run-through training post in Core Medical Training/Core Surgical Training at ST2 level and you secure an ST3 post in the local allocation stage, you are still eligible to apply for another ST3 post in the later open national competition for medical or surgical specialties.

Advantages and disadvantages of a locally-led system

Good points

- Applicants have an unlimited number of applications until they secure a post.
- Applicants can apply to an unlimited number of deaneries.
- Applicants can apply to many different specialties of their choice provided that they are eligible.

Bad points

- There is potential to have to complete many different application forms.
- There is no guarantee of an ST training post.
- Multiple deanery websites and other websites to watch and coordinate to avoid missing application deadlines.

Eligibility

There are a number of crucial criteria for being able to apply for ST, as follows.

(i) Registration with the GMC

You will need to hold full GMC registration status.

(ii) **Right to work in the UK**

UK and European Economic Area (EEA) nationals, and doctors whose immigration status entitles them to work as a doctor in training in the UK, are eligible to apply for ST posts. Evidence of immigration status would be a date-stamped passport and an accompanying letter from the Home Office. Both of these documents would need to be dated at, or prior to, the application closing date. Other non-UK or non-EEA nationals with limited leave to remain in the UK, whose employment will require a Work Permit, are subject to the resident labour market test (i.e. they would only be considered if there was no suitable UK or EEA national to fill the post).

You will be asked to bring your passport and proof of your immigration status to any interviews or assessments you attend.

(iii) **English language skills**

Applicants who completed undergraduate training in any language other than English need to provide written evidence of English language skills and will be required to bring this to any interviews or assessment centres that are attended.

(iv) **College examinations**

College examinations are not always mandatory for progression. For example, Membership of the Royal College of Physicians (MRCP) is no longer essential to allow progression from CT2 to ST3 in the medical specialties. However, you should check individual personal specifications on your local deanery website for entry at the level to which you are applying – you must have received notification of having sat and passed the exam by the closing date of your application.

(v) **Personal specification**

Each specialty has a nationally agreed 'personal specification' that lists the required competencies for that specialty. You will need to provide evidence to prove that you have achieved the specified competencies.

Before even looking at the application form, it is important to read the personal specification for the individual specialty for which you are applying. These set out the ENTRY CRITERIA and the SELECTION CRITERIA and state exactly what is essential and desirable when entering ST. It is also extremely useful to keep this nearby when completing the application form.

(vi) Match to specialty level

For entry into ST1 (specialty training year 1) and CT1 (core training year 1) levels you need to show that you have all the Foundation Programme competencies (or equivalent evidence if you have not come through this system). You must not have held a post for more than 12 months in the specialty to which you are applying.

For entry into ST2 (specialty training year 2)/CT2 (core training year 2) you will have to have achieved the equivalent of all the competencies from the first year of specialty training (ST1). However, there is no limit on experience for eligibility for selection to ST2/CT2.

For entry into specialty training years 3 and 4 (ST3/ST4) you will need to have achieved the equivalent competencies from the first 2 years of ST (ST1 and ST2). Again there is no limit on experience for eligibility.

White space answers and application scoring

Since the Tooke report, application forms now contain a combination of:

i)   Curriculum vitae (CV)-based questions (which often involve your academic achievements); and
ii) competency-based questions (which are based upon the personal specifications for each specialty).

These 'white space answers' allow the applicant to respond in prose to the question posed. There is always a word limit – for

ST applications this is often up to 150 words (for academic applications some questions go up to 250 words). When completing the form, keep to that limit to avoid any chance of being penalized. The approach to these questions is covered in detail in Section B of this book. Application scoring sheets vary from deanery to deanery. Scoring can be based on essential and desirable criteria on the application forms.

Example scoring system

In a recent academic ST3 application form, the application selection was split into a maximum score of 14 points for essential criteria and a maximum score of 22 points for desirable criteria.

Essential criteria – to achieve a maximum score

4 points: Commitment to specialty – ample clear and comprehensive evidence of commitment and clearly links experience to the post being applied for

3 points: Academic experience – evidence of above average academic experience

3 points: Clinical experience – evidence of above average clinical experience

2 points: Reasoned analytical approach – provides evidence throughout of reasons for applying

2 points: Language skills – provides clear and precise use of English

Desirable criteria – to achieve a maximum score

4 points: Key academic achievements – evidence of outstanding achievement

4 points: Scientific publications – greater than four major contributions, and at least one leading journal in that specialty

3 points: For BA/MSc/PhD or equivalent being 1st class

3 points: Scientific presentation – international presentation

2 points: Teaching experience – for a formal teaching role

2 points: Extracurricular activities – for activities that are relevant to career in specialty

2 points: Postgraduate/undergraduate prizes – three or more, or one highly prestigious prize

2 points: Honours/distinctions – for three or more of these

Other CT and ST shortlisting score sheets use the same areas to differentiate between candidates.

Other areas that could be assessed (ESSENTIAL or DESIRABLE) are:

- Experience of procedures – with above average procedural experience scoring up to 2 marks
- Evidence or participation in audits – with audits that may have been presented on a national or international stage being scored higher than just evidence of participation
- Evidence of working in multidisciplinary teams/working with others – with those showing a greater insight into this scoring higher
- Evidence of attendance at postgraduate courses such as ALS, ATLS, APLS
- Evidence of Information Technology skills – with completion of courses such as the European Computer Driving Licence (ECDL) scoring up to 2 marks (2 potentially easy marks on a score sheet!)
- Evidence of ability to work under pressure and evidence of organizational skills, which on some score sheets can gain you up to 2 marks
- In some surgical specialties, evidence of adequate progression of career, and evidence of completion of Locum Appointments for Training (LAT) posts gain extra marks.

In the 2008 applications, having passed the MRCP was NOT an essential criterion for progression from ST2/CT2 to ST3, BUT those with full membership scored an additional 2 points, offering a significant advantage over those without the examination. However, the rules relating to this may change in the future. Most applications for ST posts come with the corresponding score sheet available for scrutiny.

The interview process

After applications have been scored, the highest scoring candidates are offered interviews, with the proportion of those offered an interview being at the discretion of the deanery. The interview process may take place over a number of days or even a few weeks in large specialties and large deaneries. Typically you will hear the results of the interview after a few days.

The interview scoring and approach to the interview are discussed in Section C of this book.

- Read the personal specification and check if application forms have a shortlisting score sheet attached to them.

- Look out for the 'easy marks' to score or lose out on – such as gaining the European Computer Driving Licence (ECDL), ensuring the appropriate use of English language, etc. If you miss out on these, you may miss out on being shortlisted for interviews.

- Ensure that you check your eligibility before applying and have gained the appropriate competencies, so that administration issues do not prevent your progression.

4 Dissecting the application process

Philip J Smith, Manoj Ramachandran and Marc A Gladman

Specialty training themes

There are a number of main themes within the specialty training (ST) application process that are covered to a variable extent in the application forms and interviews.

- Lifelong learning: past, present and future – this relates to your academic achievements, research and audit experience, and your teaching skills – these are independently assessed both within your application form and interview. Furthermore, a crucial aspect is your grasp of clinical governance and other current NHS issues (e.g. control of hospital-acquired infection).
- Professional behaviour/non-clinical skills – possibly the most important part of the application process. Your professional integrity and ability to implement good medical practice will be assessed together with your non-clinical skills (teamwork, leadership, etc.).
- Clinical skills – these are particularly assessed at the interview. Expect to undergo a mini clinical examination style viva, where you will be cross-questioned to establish your ability to cope under pressure, to prioritize clinical care and to keep the patient as the central focus of care. Often this is assessed in the form of clinical scenarios.

Realistic expectations for specialty training

Recent years have seen unprecedented levels of competition for training places in the UK, especially with the implementation of ST replacing the old system of training. However, a degree of competition has always been present, even in the 'old system' of training rotations. Furthermore, there have always been specialties that are more sought after than others (e.g. plastic surgery and cardiology at ST3 entry). By contrast, audiological medicine may not be as oversubscribed by applicants, but you have to bear in mind that the number of positions available in such a specialty will be very limited. In real terms, this may lead to a similar ratio of competition of jobs to applicants.

Geographical location is also important, as competition within the same specialty may be vastly different from deanery to deanery, since some deaneries may have more applicants but fewer vacancies and vice versa. Therefore, you need to decide at an early stage whether location or specialty is more important. In the case of the former, if you are desperate to work in a particular area of the country, you may wish to consider applying for a less competitive specialty (but ensure that it is one that you will still enjoy doing for the rest of your life!) in your preferred deanery. Remember, however, you are applying to a deanery and some deaneries cover very large geographical areas. On the other hand, if you are totally committed to working in only one specialty, you may have to consider applying to deaneries that are less competitive for your chosen specialty.

Most deaneries now publish competition ratios for the individual specialties on their websites. You must examine these before applying for the ST job you want, as it will give you an idea of what you are up against in pursuit of your dream job.

Clearly, the best applicants get the best jobs in the best places. Therefore, your application form and performance at interview need to be flawless. This book aims to help you prepare as much as possible so that you can excel. Ultimately, however, you need to reflect on your own abilities and strengths before you apply, and where your priorities lie. It sounds quite deep, but in the world of run-through training, the design is such that you 'run' with the programme and don't look back – so the decisions you make are big ones! If you want to apply to a specialty because you would regret it if you didn't, then you should, but with your eyes open and with realistic expectation, rather than blind hope!

Application form format

Recent application forms for ST have reverted to being very similar in appearance to the 'old' style forms used for Specialist Registrar (SpR) applications from a few years ago. They are typically divided up into the following sections.

Section A: Personal details

Details asked for usually include: name, address, date of birth, address for correspondence, date available to start post if offered.

Section B: General Medical Council (GMC) registration

Details asked for usually include: type of registration, GMC number, renewal date and name in which you are registered.

Section C: Professional qualifications

Details asked for usually include: university/medical school attended, with dates of study.

These sections typically do not constitute part of the scoring but are important for eligibility and ENTRY CRITERIA, which depending on your specialty and stage in career include evidence of: eligibility for registration with the GMC, university qualifications, eligibility to work in the UK, evidence of previous Foundation or ST competencies, the correct amount of time experience in the specialty you are applying for (this will be stated on the personal specification for the job).

Section D: Further professional qualifications

You may be asked to complete a table like this:

Degree/diploma (state class of degree awarded)	Awarding body	Date of qualification
BSc Immunology (1st class)	University of London	07/07/2004
MBBS (Distinction)	University of London	07/07/2006

In this table you would also include any previous degrees and higher degrees (such as MSc/PhD), as well as qualifications such as MRCP, MRCS, and so on.

Sections E and F: Current and past employment

This section is important as the selectors will decide whether you are eligible for entry in that current specialty and at the particular level that you are applying for. This information may also need to be tabulated, listing the specialty, hospital and consultant you worked for. It may also ask for start and finishing dates, and length of contracts. It may even ask you whether these are training or non-training posts and their grades. It is best to list them in chronological order.

Section G: Procedural skills

You may be asked to list the clinical procedures that you have performed and then list your competency in them.

Be cautious when completing this section and do not lie. There is no point saying that you are highly experienced in placing temporary pacing wires as an F2 doctor if you are not, as the selectors are unlikely to believe you!

Sections H, I, J, K, L, M

These sections cover the 'white space' questions related to audit, management skills, communication skills, initiative, teaching, research and commitment to specialty. Completion of such questions will be covered in detail in the subsequent sections of this book.

Remaining sections

You will most probably be asked to list your publications, presentations, posters, prizes and other honours. This seems straightforward, but you should always:

- Ensure that they are listed in chronological order.
- If citing a publication ensure that you cite them correctly as they would be cited on PubMed.
- If listing a presentation or poster remember to state whether they were at local, national or international conferences, and list what you were presenting, where, and when.
- If listing your prizes, honours and other achievements, such as a University Gold Award, ensure that you state what the prize was, who awarded it and when it was awarded.

On most applications you will be asked to list two referees – usually this is your current consultant or educational supervisor, plus another consultant of your choosing. These should be two consultants that you have worked for before.

5 How to get THAT job: an insider's guide

Marc A Gladman and Manoj Ramachandran

'You have decided that you want to be a cardiologist. It is the only specialty for you. But you are concerned by the anticipated competition for training posts. So, is it time to switch to plan B (general practice) and play it safe, as has been suggested?'

Heard S. Choosing your hospital specialty. *BMJ Career Focus* 2006; 332: 221

Fortune favours the brave

Well, perhaps not just yet. You will spend at least the next 40 years working in your chosen specialty – a long time to be unhappy if you choose one in which you have little or no interest. Choosing a pathway that will provide job satisfaction is crucial and should be based primarily on your interests and aspirations, the level of skills that you possess and your (realistic) chances of getting the job. It should not be based around tactical workforce planning or fear of competition. If there are only 'x' posts available in 'cardiology', ask yourself not 'what should I do instead?' but 'what do I have to do to secure one of them?'. Stay positive and consider your options carefully before deciding whether you ought to compromise your choice. In this chapter, we will help you prepare yourself for the application process, and most importantly, provide you with some important information about how best to 'sell yourself' to maximize your chances of getting appointed.

Remember
Your MOST important objective during the application process is to demonstrate an 'edge' over the competition, so that you stand out from the crowd.

Sell yourself

To stand out from the crowd you MUST be prepared to *sell yourself*. Most doctors are uncomfortable with this concept, as we are not used to doing it and receive little or no instruction on how to achieve it. During the application process, the selectors are seeking evidence of specific academic achievements and clinical and non-clinical skills.

It may sound obvious, but unless you adequately demonstrate (and communicate to the selectors!) satisfactory attainment of the skills sought in the application process you will not pick up the points on offer and thus you will not get appointed.

At first consideration, you may not appreciate that you possess some of these skills that are being sought. Consequently, you must allow yourself appropriate time to sit down and carefully scrutinize your curriculum vitae (CV) and extracurricular achievements. The questions posed are aimed at evaluating your personal skills, attributes and characteristics. These are required of specialty trainees and you will have invariably started to develop them in the Foundation or Core Training Programmes. However, you may have to search long and deep to identify them!

Avoid appearing self-effacing or undervaluing your own achievements for the sake of modesty. Remember, this application is YOUR sales pitch. Only YOU can sell yourself.

However, while you must sell your strengths, the importance of humility cannot be overstated, particularly as the selectors will be senior to you!

All doctors are equal ... but some are more equal than others

Selection for specialty training (ST) posts involves the assessment of numerous clinical and non-clinical skills. The importance of clinical skills in facilitating career progression need not be emphasized and must be demonstrated in the application process. Even if you consider yourself to be the greatest diagnostician that ever practiced medicine, you are unlikely to be able to demonstrate your clinical acumen on an application form. This leaves academic achievements and non-clinical skills (e.g. leadership, motivation, communication, teaching, etc.) as the variables that differentiate between candidates. They are thus employed as discriminators to determine 'who gets the job'. As it is usually too late to boost your academic achievements in the few weeks prior to applying for an ST post, optimum demonstration and adequate communication of your non-clinical skills is your best opportunity to maximize your overall score.

Securing an ST post: the three Ss of success

Competition for ST posts can be fierce, particularly in certain regions of the country. In addition to ensuring that you score highly enough to gain entry to your desired ST Programme, maximizing your score is crucial in ensuring that you get the actual rotation that you want within the deanery to which you are appointed. Remember, someone has to get that job ... but will it be *you*? When you sit down to start thinking about applying for an ST post, we suggest that you consider the three Ss to optimize your chance of success.

The three Ss of success

- Self-awareness

- Strategy

- Score maximization

Self-awareness

Remember to take some time out to think about where and what you are applying for and what your realistic goals are. Before you apply, you need to decide:

- Which specialty interests you and how much do you want to do it?
- What relevant experience/aptitude do you have for this specialty?

There are some key questions that you must ask of yourself, in an attempt to objectively appraise your own abilities/chances.

- Do you meet the personal specification?
- Where do your strengths lie?
- How competitive do you feel you will be, based on your CV and other skills – just how good are you compared with your peers?
- What are your most significant clinical/academic/non-clinical achievements to date?
- Do you have any achievements that are unique to you?
- Can you communicate these facts *effectively* on the application form and at interview?

Careful consideration of these questions will enable you to determine if you are likely to succeed in getting appointed – what are your career prospects *realistically*? Do you deserve *that* job in *that* location? It is often useful to enlist the help of your immediate seniors and/or your educational supervisor to gain a more objective opinion.

List the skills/aptitudes necessary for your chosen specialty.

List the ways in which you have demonstrated aptitude for your chosen specialty, e.g. attendance at scientific meetings, additional specialist outpatient clinics, skills courses, etc.

Strategy

Strategy for applying

Having established an idea of your 'chances', the next crucial step is to decide on a strategy for applying for ST posts. Key considerations here that will require a variable degree of research are set out below.

- At which level of ST entry are you most suited/competitive?
- How many posts are available in your chosen specialty?
- How popular is your chosen specialty?
- How popular is the deanery to which you will be applying?
- Is your chosen specialty any less competitive in other deaneries?

Ultimately, you need to decide which is most important to you – location or specialty? Establish your job priorities – are you willing to compromise location or specialty, or both, to secure an ST post? Selecting a correct strategy for application determines your chances of getting shortlisted and then appointed. Remember that only the *best* applicants will secure jobs in *competitive* specialties in *popular* locations. Tailor your application accordingly. It is also important to ensure that you are familiar with the format of the application forms and interviews, and the themes within them. Be sure to leave yourself enough time to complete the form and prepare for the interview. This will require that you are familiar with the timeframe for application and keep this in mind when planning social activities. Finally, remember that there are NO limits to the number of jobs that you can apply for, re-utilization of most of the information on your forms can be used for multiple applications. However, if you are not getting shortlisted your application form is inadequate in some way, so there is no point in re-using it!

Strategy for completing the application form/preparing for interview

When beginning to tackle your form, consider the **five Ps**.

The five Ps

- **Prepare** your material – have the questions and personal specifications available

- **Pensive** – think long and hard for the best and most original example

- **Plan** – how you will structure your answers

- **Produce** a draft – this will (dramatically!) exceed the word count

- **Perfect** – reduce to comply with word count; check grammar and syntax

Remember, the questions on the application form and those asked at interview are usually repeated each year. Get ahead of the competition by starting your preparation well in advance. Those around you may appear to be blasé about their application, but rest assured that, privately, they will be taking it very seriously. Remember, you are in direct competition with your peers. Once the post is advertised, cancel holidays, lock yourself away, and concentrate only on your application. Time is short once the process begins. You should aim to perfect your answers so that not a single word is wasted. The first, early drafts will almost certainly be well over the word limit and needlessly wordy. Each subsequent draft should improve on the last until every single available point is picked up. You should aim to redraft each answer at least 5–10 times.

- **The form and preparing for interview WILL take longer to complete than you envisage – do NOT leave it until the night before!**

- **The form WILL need amending/require several drafts.**

- **You WILL make basic errors – use a spell check and get trusted friends and colleagues to proofread for errors of syntax and grammar.**

Score maximization

Scoring of application form responses

Wouldn't it be easier to secure an ST post if you knew in advance how the selectors score your application form and performance at interview? For the application form at least, details of the marks available for individual questions are usually provided in the application pack. Obviously, the details of exactly how, and for what, these marks are allocated within individual questions are confidential. It would be inappropriate, therefore, for any specific details relating to this to be divulged. Furthermore, the marking scheme varies from deanery to deanery and from year to year. That said, it is important to appreciate that the scorers will be looking out for certain indicators when marking your responses. Some (desirable factors) will increase your score, whilst others (undesirable factors) will decrease your score. The relative proportion of each of these factors will determine your overall score. The obvious aim is to provide the scorers with as many of the desirable and as few of the undesirable factors as possible to maximize your score for each question.

What are the selectors looking for and how can you give them what they want?

- The skills/attributes that you need to demonstrate to the selectors that you possess can be found in the personal specification for the ST post.

- Print off the personal specification and have it in front of you as you complete the application form. Cross off each skill/attribute as you go and ensure that you have demonstrated ALL of them somewhere in your responses!

As previously mentioned in Chapter 4, the majority of marks on offer in the application form are assessed in 'white space' questions related to audit, management skills, communication skills, initiative, teaching, research, commitment to specialty, etc. Similarly, these topics will also be assessed and scored at interview.

Therefore, you must have a reliable approach to answering such questions. Commonly, we find that (otherwise good) applicants perform least well when answering these questions, exploring your non-clinical skills.

- **The significance of non-clinical skills is frequently overlooked by applicants, leading to crucial points being 'dropped'.**

- **The most common mistake that applicants make during the application process is to put far too much emphasis on describing medical facts (demonstrating clinical skills) when answering questions that are seeking to establish the satisfactory attainment of non-clinical skills (e.g. leadership, teamwork, motivation, etc.).**

- **A classic example of this is when applicants describe a trauma/arrest call when answering a teamwork question and proceed to consume all of the available word count in describing the clinical scenario (patient's vital signs, drugs/fluids administered, etc.), rather than the actions that demonstrate the ability to function as part of a team (allocation of tasks, identification of roles within the team, control of team members, appraisal of individual/team performance, etc.).**

Demonstrate a competitive edge: 'unique selling points' (USPs) and 'BIG GUNS'

Demonstration of a *'career edge'* that sets you apart from the competition is crucial. We recommend careful scrutiny of your clinical and (more importantly) non-clinical achievements to date to identify your USPs. These are your most significant achievements that make you stand out from the crowd and that are unique to you. These will form your **'BIG GUNS'** that you will use to demonstrate to the selectors that they should appoint *YOU!*

- In addition to printing off the personal specification for your ST post, you should have your USPs in front of you when you complete your application form and prepare for the interview.
- These 'big guns' will form the basis of the example that you describe to demonstrate that you possess the skills/attributes that the selectors are looking for in that particular question.
- For example: if your 'big gun' was completing a research project and obtaining a publication during your elective, this would demonstrate the following skills (and many others not provided here!): ability to set goals, prioritize, multi-task, manage your time efficiently, etc. Thus, this big gun could be used as the scenario in questions asking you to demonstrate your organization skills.

At first glance, you may feel that you haven't achieved anything worthy or unique enough to use. This is where you need to invest time in really thinking about all the things that you have done in your career, often without realizing their significance at the time.

Q: What are some typical examples of USPs/big guns?

A: Clearly, it is impossible for anyone other than YOU to identify YOUR USPs. Your 'big guns' should be things that you have done that are *over* and *above* what many others will have done or what is expected of you in the day-to-day job. Suitable examples might include:

- Raising money for a local charity by completing a particular task
- Organizing a particular event that turned out to be a notable success
- Attendance at scientific meetings related to your specialty.

Q: What should I NOT use as USPs/big guns?

A: Avoid using things that are simply *expected* duties of your job. For example:

- Practical procedures (e.g. central line insertion)
- Collecting morbidity/mortality data for the weekly surgical audit meetings
- Teaching medical students.

If you are *not* doing these things, you are not doing your job!

List your most significant achievements that make you stand out from the crowd and that are unique to you; the key points that you want to get across to the selectors *at all costs*. These will form your 'big guns' that you should use when answering white space and interview questions. Completion of this section is crucial and you should keep your responses to hand when completing the application form and while preparing for the interview.

 List your most significant clinical/academic achievements.

List your most significant clinical/academic/non-clinical achievements.

What skills does each of your big guns demonstrate?

Approach to individual questions on the form

There are some key considerations when preparing your responses. These will be addressed in turn.

Read the question and answer everything that is asked

Answer *exactly* what the question is asking, and do not be tempted to answer a different question. This sounds obvious, but all too often, applicants write the response to a question they wished they had been asked rather than the one that was actually asked! It is often helpful when planning your response to break the question down into its constituent parts. For example:

Give one example of a non-academic achievement explaining both the significance to you and the relevance to specialty training.

This question can be broken down into

(i)   One example of a *non-academic* achievement
(ii) Its significance to *you*
(iii) Its *relevance* to ST.

Choose your examples like a 'PRO'

The questions on the form are seeking to determine whether you possess specific skills/qualities required of specialty trainees, as set out in the personal specification document. For example, if you are asked to provide an example of teamworking, really try to identify one specific example that both requires a team approach and demonstrates your ability to work in a team. You must avoid the temptation to talk about your general experience when asked to give *specific* examples. Examples with clearly defined outcomes tend to work better, particularly those that have a positive outcome. Make sure that you incorporate your BIG GUNS wherever possible.

The examples that you choose for each of the questions should satisfy the **PRO** criteria.

Act like a PRO

- **Personal** – delve into your personal experience.

- **Relevant** – it must demonstrate the skill/quality being sought in the question.

- **Original** – come up with something that won't be used by your peers (competitors!). This is your chance to impress the marker.

Examples to avoid at all costs are those that:

- **Many others will use, e.g. multidisciplinary or cardiac arrest teams for teamworking questions.**

- **Are too negative or attribute blame to others.**

- **Are above your level of medical experience, e.g. an ST1 doctor would not be expected to operate on a patient with a ruptured abdominal aortic aneurysm!**

Be precise and concise, correct your spelling and use 'power verbs'

The number of words that you are allowed to use for each of your responses is limited on the form. Many applicants see this as a disadvantage, but it actually encourages the construction of concise sentences. However, ensure that you precisely provide responses to each component of the question. There is no excuse for grammatical errors or spelling mistakes when completing the form. Your response may be marked down for such errors. Computer spell checks are not always accurate or sufficient; get your finished article proofread by someone else.

Passive descriptions will have far less impact than the use of active or 'power' verbs when used in a sentence. Power verbs such as 'accomplished', 'negotiated' and 'facilitated' will give your sentences a great deal more impact than 'completed', 'arranged' and 'helped'.

A selection of power verbs

Accomplished	Analysed	Coordinated
Designed	Directed	Designated
Established	Evaluated	Facilitated
Formulated	Implemented	Instigated
Negotiated	Organized	Prioritized
Scheduled	Supervised	Validated

Use a structure such as the SPAR technique

A clear structure to your answer is essential. A well-structured answer not only makes identification of key points easier for the markers, guaranteeing that you receive all the marks that you deserve, but also ensures that you address, and thus score points, for *every* section of the question. We advocate the use of the acronym **SPAR** for this purpose.

The SPAR technique

- **S**ituation
- **P**roblem
- **A**ction
- **R**esult/**R**eflection/**R**elevance to ST

Situation

The situation sets the scene for the rest of the answer and details your chosen example. You should very briefly but *clearly* describe your example, keeping it relevant to the question. The description should be precise and concise and should focus only on those details that are pertinent to your answer. Avoid waffling as this creates a bad first impression and consumes words that will be needed later on.

Problem

Having succinctly described your example, it is useful to define a specific problem that needed to be addressed. Together with the situation above, this section should account for approximately one-third of the word allocation.

Action

This section describes what YOU did. Usually, this section accounts for approximately one-third of the word allocation. You should concentrate on demonstrating those personal skills/attributes/characteristics that are required of an ST doctor, as set out in the personal specification. Consider what actions/power verbs describe the clinical/personal skill being evaluated (e.g. teamworking), rather than simply keep mentioning that skill!

Result/reflection/relevance to specialty training

Ideally, your example should have a positive and definite outcome that can be described accurately. Try to draw relevant conclusions from the example. More importantly, marks are available for reflecting on what you have learnt and how this knowledge is relevant and applicable to ST. Omission of these last two elements is the main reason for applicants to drop marks – address them in every question to maximize the marks that you are awarded.

Tell the truth

DO NOT be tempted to fabricate examples or embellish them to make them sound more impressive. Likewise, exaggerating your role in any given situation should be avoided. Don't forget that one of the scorers will be a medical doctor, who will be fully aware of what is appropriate for your level of training. Anyone even suspected of submitting an invalid or falsified response will have their application referred on to the chief assessor, who may then lead on to referral to the central authorities.

Q: What are the most crucial considerations to ensure that I achieve high scores for my responses?

A: You must:

- Provide clear and relevant examples
- Demonstrate clear evidence of reflection/learning
- Appreciate how your experience will be relevant to ST.

Q: What annoys the scorers the most and will result in me achieving poor scores?

A: They get most annoyed by:

- Spelling and grammatical mistakes
- Using poor or irrelevant examples
- Spending too much time on and too many words describing the example
- A lack of learning/reflection from the situation
- Failure to explain the relevance to ST.

Q: How can I use all the tips provided in this chapter to construct a sample answer?

A: Complete in steps as follows:

1. Identify your 'big guns'.

2. Read the question on the application form and cross-check with the personal specification to see which skills are being sought.

3. Select the 'big gun' that is most pertinent to the question being asked, ensuring that it meets the PRO criteria.

4. Use the SPAR technique to answer the question.

Worked example:

1. Big guns: completing a research project and obtaining a publication during your elective; raising £6000 for a local charity; attendance at the international annual meeting of cardiologists.

2. Question on application form: provide an example of an achievement that demonstrates your organization skills.

3. Select the most appropriate big gun for this question: raising £6000 for a local charity, demonstrating the following organization skills, i.e. ability to set goals, prioritize, multi-task, manage your time efficiently, etc.

4. Application of SPAR:

[Situation and problem]

I initiated and managed an 'aerobics marathon' in central London to increase awareness about homeless dogs.

[Actions]

In advance, I listed all the important tasks that needed to be completed (demonstrates goal setting). I prioritized these tasks, identifying that hire of the aerobics machines was the most crucial consideration (demonstrates ability to prioritize). Before the event, I simultaneously arranged the hire of all necessary equipment and for 30 friends to offer their services over a 12-hour period to keep the aerobics machines running and to collect money from the general public (demonstrating multi-tasking and completion on time). The day before the event, I was informed that there would be no rowing machines available for hire and thus I elected to use cross-trainers instead (demonstrating the ability to form contingency plans under pressure).

[Result/reflection]

I successfully raised in excess of £6000 for the Save Every Single Dog Fund and as a consequence I have improved my ability to communicate clearly and to achieve complex tasks outside of a medical environment. I also learned to prioritize my tasks whilst ensuring that they are all completed efficiently.

Golden tips for a successful application

- Set aside plenty of time to prepare and construct your answers.

- Complete the application form in stages.

- Always read the question carefully and highlight keywords.

- Select your examples carefully – consider which example will display your skills best. Use your BIG GUNS!!

- Avoid repetition and do not use the same example twice.

- Ensure that you answer every part of the question.

- Be concise and keep within the word limit.

- Proofread your answers.

- Check for mistakes in spelling and grammar.

- Print yourself a hard copy and recheck it.

- Submit your application form as early as possible to allow for any glitches.

- Breathe a huge sigh of relief and relax!

SECTION B
Completing the application form

6 Academic achievements

Luke Moore and Philip J Smith

Academic activities primarily involve three facets of our practice – education, research and personal development. Each of us will have pursued academic achievements to varying levels, initially as undergraduates and now subsequently in our continuing postgraduate careers.

As each of us strives for excellence, our responses to questions on our academic achievements must portray our efforts in these wide ranges of activities. Depending on whether a candidate is applying for a *Clinical* Specialty Training scheme or an *Academic* Clinical Fellowship, the emphasis on academic achievement will vary, but questions usually cover the main topics of:

- Prizes or awards
- Publications in peer-reviewed journals
- Presentations and posters at conferences
- Research, whether past or in progress
- Teaching experience and training in teaching.

Prizes, publications and presentations usually require simple lists. For the majority of applications, the academic section is broken down into these sub-questions, but occasionally a synoptic question is posed, which requires you to actively mention each of these components within your answer.

To score top marks, you should not only show that you have experience of these activities, but also be able to reflect upon how these have developed your abilities and how they will lead to further academic accomplishments.

There are several avenues you can pursue as a postgraduate to further your academic credentials, some of them involve a reasonable amount of work, so be prepared!

Ways to boost your academic achievements

- Postgraduate diplomas – these show that you not only have a vested interest in the specialty but also have the initiative to advance your knowledge/skills in this area and the stamina to carry this through. Examples of areas that have both distance and taught diplomas include: tropical medicine, medical education (and surgical education), public health, HIV, trauma surgery ... the list goes on.

- Specialty essays – again these not only show your commitment to a specialty, but often lead to presentations and publications. Numerous institutions offer (usually eponymous) essay prizes including: the Royal College of Physicians (Teale), Royal Society of Medicine (a plethora), Royal College of Psychiatry (Gaskell, President's), etc.

- Short courses – many short courses are available to improve generic academic skills. These include: Good Clinical Practice, Research Governance, Teaching the Teachers, Critical Analysis, Clinical Statistics & Epidemiology.

- Get involved with medical schools – contacting your local undergraduate department can lead to fruitful time spent facilitating, examining, tutoring, etc. undergraduates, which all boost your education experience.

- Take every opportunity to publish – original research projects are extremely difficult to get off the ground in your early postgraduate years. Don't let this deter you – general interest/observational articles/published audits still have a place.

- Don't make up prizes/articles/lectures/presentations!

- Don't leave a box blank – search your curriculum vitae (CV) and find something, anything, to put in each section.

- Don't be passive – cast your role in an active and positive light.

- Remember that you are the one applying – state your level of participation in any projects as 'I' rather than 'we'.

- Don't just state events – mention the skills you brought to the project (such as initiative, enthusiasm, analytical skills) and those gained from your involvement (understanding of Good Clinical Practice/Research Governance, appreciation of the role of the Research & Ethics Committee, etc.).

- Make sure you show *continuing* academic achievement throughout your undergraduate and postgraduate career.

Lists

As we discussed earlier, several sections within the academic achievement section will require lists of your accomplishments. This is usually a quick and simple area of the form but it is important to remember some fundamental rules.

- Never use abbreviations – you might understand exactly what you mean and think that everyone else should too, but abbreviations confuse and irritate those not in the know (e.g. your selector!).

List your presentations.

Poor answer

Presentations/posters at conferences

HIV and 4G NPTs in the NHS. Bloggs S, Jones M.

Presented at the RSTMH National Annual Conference July 2008.

This example was taken from an Academic Clinical Fellowship application form, and demonstrates how irritating abbreviations are!

Better answer

Presentations/posters at conferences

*Human Immunodeficiency Virus and Fourth Generation Near Patient Tests in the National Health Service. **Bloggs S**, Jones M. Annual Meeting of Immunologists, London, June 2009.*

Presented at the Royal Society of Tropical Medicine & Hygiene National Annual Conference July 2008.

Bold your name – it will help to orientate the assessor to your role in the project. Above and beyond this, some application forms ask for clarification of your specific role in a project.

If you have undertaken or are undertaking a research project, please give details and indicate your involvement.

Poor answer

Bond C, Moore L, Roberts C. Accuracy of Clinician Diagnoses of COPD in the Elderly.

Project initiated at Professorial level, with registrar support. I was integrally involved in data collection, consenting for participation in the research and organizing ethical approval

Better answer

*Bond C, **Moore L**, Roberts C. Accuracy of Clinician Diagnoses of COPD in the Elderly.*

Acted as primary data collector and undertook active roles in obtaining Research & Ethics Committee approval and independent funding. Obtained professorial supervision and work currently submitted for peer review.

Golden tips for a successful application

- Cite published references correctly – the standard accepted manner is using the Vancouver style – do not deviate.

- Cite publications in chronological order – the most recent first – and if the question asks for a specific piece of information, such as the PubMed number, be sure to include it!

- Use bolding appropriately, not excessively!

Please list your publications with full citation and PubMed number. Please asterisk those for which you are first author.

Poor answer

Bond C, Moore L, Roberts C. Accuracy of Clinician Diagnoses of COPD in the Elderly. *Age Aging. Oct 2006;301:244-9.*

Moore L *et al.* Effects of exercise in the rehabilitation of elderly patients with COPD. Arch Gerontol Geriatr. *2008 Mar-Apr;28(2):31-8.*

Better answer

* **Moore L**, Kyu Tun J, Wadhwani S. Effects of exercise in the rehabilitation of elderly patients with COPD. *Arch Gerontol Geriatr.* 2008;28(2):31-8. PMID: 18656098

Bond C, **Moore L**, Roberts C. Accuracy of Clinician Diagnoses of COPD in the Elderly. *Age Aging* 2006;301:244-9. PMID:18875443

Open questions

It is a bit more difficult to answer generic open academic questions. Remember to include with each point (i) a description of what you did, (ii) what you gained from the experience and (iii) how you are going to take this forward.

In what way have you pursued an academic role in your career so far? (150 words)

Poor answer

I graduated from the University of Leeds in 2003 and always did well throughout medical school. Between my third year and my fourth year I undertook an intercalated BSc in Biochemistry. During my BSc I was given a laboratory based project from which I published an article. After graduating I have continued to publish – one of my consultants recently suggested we write an article on an interesting case that we had – I was second author in this article. I am thinking about undertaking the Diploma of Tropical Medicine & Hygiene because I am interested in doing some voluntary work overseas. I am also very interested in teaching, particularly in teaching medical students, and always go out of my way to teach them procedures. At my ARCP it was suggested I book myself onto a teaching course which I have now completed.

Better answer

As an academic undergraduate, I achieved an intercalated First-class degree in Neuroscience from which I obtained a publication from my dissertation in a peer-reviewed journal. This developed my knowledge of research methodology and enabled me to exert autonomy and display initiative. As a postgraduate, I organised and successfully completed the Diploma in Neurology, gaining analytical skills and insight into research techniques. I have continued to publish, winning the McGovern prize for my peer-reviewed essay on multiple sclerosis. Recently, I have submitted an audit that altered Trust policy for publication. Currently, I am developing a research protocol investigating molecular factors implicated in multiple sclerosis that I intend to complete as part of a higher degree. I am also actively involved in teaching, having completed the Teaching the Teachers course. I have applied the methods in tutoring undergraduates & junior doctors in practice and also in my role as a facilitator for undergraduates at University College London.

Analysis

The two example answers above portray similar academic histories, but described in increasingly attractive ways. The emphasis shifts from initially just documenting details of the achievements themselves to what the achievements provided in terms of personal attributes and academic skills. There is also a subtle shift in the emphasis on the drive behind the experiences. The 'poor answer' reflects how the candidate relied upon others to formulate their academic credentials. The latter, better answer shows initiative and enthusiasm, it also briefly outlines the applicant's current activities whilst touching on plans for the future – points like this can provide useful building blocks for discussion in the interview.

If you have undertaken or are undertaking a research project, please give details and indicate your involvement.

- Before you start, sit down and pick out all the academic achievements you have so far from your CV.

- Remember the common pitfalls.

- Don't just list your achievements – reflect upon them.

- Answer the question!

- Stick to the word limit.

- There is a fine line between buzzwords and superfluous words.

7 Teaching and learning

Jasdeep Gill and Sukhjinder Nijjer

Introduction

Among the numerous roles and responsibilities of a doctor, teaching and learning are high on the priority list. This is by no means a recent recognition, and was identified within the Hippocratic Oath many years ago. However, in recent years, the teaching and learning needs of doctors have moved up the agenda and transformed the way in which doctors train and practise.

Commitment to lifelong learning is an essential element of being professionally qualified. The Department of Health has introduced a lifelong learning framework, which primarily aims to support NHS staff to acquire new skills and to ensure that patients benefit from a better qualified and more motivated workforce. Continuing professional development is considered the process of lifelong learning in practice. It includes regularly updating medical, managerial, social and personal skills to aid the multidisciplinary context of patient care. Continuing professional development is also fundamental to career progression, particularly given the passing of the concept of a 'job for life' and redefined career pathways.

The Royal Colleges, the Postgraduate Medical Education and Training Board and the General Medical Council (GMC) all recognize teaching and learning as essential parts of good medical practice as a doctor. It is therefore no surprise that demonstrating your teaching and learning abilities forms a fundamental part of the recruitment process to enter specialty training (ST).

Commitment to lifelong learning and the ability to demonstrate your abilities on the application form are vital skills that will serve you and your future patients. This chapter will discuss teaching and learning styles and how to tackle these questions using worked examples. You may have already developed certain teaching and learning styles, some of which are effective, but others less so. We will discuss several teaching and learning methods that may help stimulate ideas for answers on your application form.

Teaching and learning styles

The introduction of competency-based training and learning portfolios further emphasizes the drive of lifelong learning. However, it also demonstrates the shift from the 'teacher as expert', which involved a didactic teaching approach, to the 'teacher as facilitator', which involves a teacher guiding the learner towards sources of knowledge so that the learner discovers the answer. Teaching styles that support this approach include problem-based learning (PBL), self-directed learning (SDL) and discussion. From the descriptions below, try to identify which is the predominant teaching style for you.

Didactic/direct instruction

This is the traditional teacher-centred approach. The teacher provides the learner with the majority of information required, often via lectures. This style allows minimal teacher–learner interaction and requires supplementation by examples, practice and discussion to check understanding.

Problem-based learning

This involves learning through structured exploration of a research problem. Learners work in small groups to define, carry out and reflect upon a research task, which can often be a 'real-life' scenario, using a systematic approach. The teacher acts as a facilitator to whom the learner can turn for guidance.

Discussion

This involves interactive and free dialogue between the teacher and learner. It involves more than simply a question and answer period, because it requires the teacher to give control to the learner(s) to express their thoughts. It requires open-mindedness and mutual respect between the teacher and learner.

Self-directed learning/self-directed instruction

This is a learner-centred approach. It allows learners to take responsibility for their own learning by applying their knowledge to real scenarios, monitoring their own achievements and exploring sources for further information. It encourages the learner to apply independent thought and enhances the development of reasoning, judgement and critical thinking skills.

Overview

Most teaching and learning interactions involve more than one style.

The teacher–learner relationship has an immense impact on the quality of teaching and learning. It is an advantage for you to recognize and use the different styles when teaching to help you meet the students' needs.

Teaching is a difficult skill to master and using the wrong approach can waste time and dishearten both yourself and the learner. Employers are keen that you have had formal training in teaching. For example, if you are assigned a regular undergraduate group to teach weekly, it would be prudent for you to have attended a course in teaching. Online and distance learning courses are available. Employers will want to see evidence of attendance and completion of these courses – essential for your portfolio on interview day.

Maintaining good learning and teaching practices not only helps you in your day-to-day role as a doctor, but is also an excellent curriculum vitae (CV) builder. Employees are keen to see your skills in teaching, appraisal and mentorship, and so the ST application questions will ask for specific examples of your ability or experience in this particular area. This style of questioning is known as competency-based questioning. Competency-based questions allow candidates to demonstrate the skills they possess that are necessary for a particular job.

When answering competency-based questions, it is better to use specific examples rather than to write broadly about your general experiences.

With lifelong learning and continuing professional development being so high up on the health-care agenda, there is no doubt that there will be questions relating to your teaching experience on the ST application. In the paragraphs that follow, there are some worked examples of ST application questions. Each question has been broken down and answered twice, first with an example of a poor answer and then with an example of a better answer using the **SPAR** technique (see Chapter 5) where applicable.

Describe one example of a teaching session that you conducted and the teaching style you used.

Poor answer

During summer this year I taught a group of house officers suturing skills. They had identified that this was a topic they wished to learn about. I had attended suturing sessions at the Royal College during my job in Orthopaedics which I found to be useful and wanted to pass on the skills I had learnt.

I booked a clinical skills room and organized the equipment required for the practical part of the teaching session. I talked them through the principles of suturing using a Powerpoint presentation and then supervised them while they practised.

They provided positive feedback and approved of my teaching technique. I refreshed and enhanced my suturing skills, which will be useful.

This answer is superficial and waffles at the start. It describes how the teaching was done but demonstrates that the candidate does not have insight into teaching styles. The final sentence correctly reflects on what the candidate has learnt; however, it demonstrates that the candidate has misidentified the point of this question.

Better answer

I taught health education to classes of 12–14-year-olds with a colleague. The school identified the curriculum, which included physical, mental and sexual health topics.

I used a mixture of didactic teaching alongside discussion and self-directed learning, which created a balance and maintained the students' interest. I encouraged student participation and for them to ask questions as I went along.

This experience significantly increased my confidence in public speaking and dealing with different age groups. I will demonstrate these skills during my specialty training and when managing and educating patients.

This answer covers each component of the question and works through the SPAR approach. The use of buzzwords such as 'didactic' and 'self-directed learning' illustrates that the candidate has knowledge of teaching styles. The answer demonstrates that the candidate recognizes teaching as a fundamental component of patient care.

- This question has many parts, so start off by breaking it down and highlighting the keywords. Notably this question is about *teaching, teaching styles* and *your* experience of teaching.

- To complete the question it asks for your *reflection* on what you have learnt and its application to your subsequent training. Even if the question did not directly ask for this, you should aim to complete your answer with a sentence or two of reflection.

- Always keep referring back to the question as you write your answer to ensure that you answer each component of the question.

Move on next to think about potential examples of teaching that you could use. This could be in relation to your medical training or from any other experience. For example, teaching medical students in lower years (e.g. Objective Structured Clinical Examination (OSCE) skills, clinical skills, basic life support classes), teaching children in schools (e.g. health education) or teaching in any extracurricular area that you are skilled in (e.g. sports, cookery, dance, etc.). Whichever example you use, be clear and concise in your description of the example. Remember you will be marked on how you taught and your experience rather than exactly who and what you taught. Aim to show some insight into why you used the teaching methods you chose. When teaching any audience or group, feedback is always a useful component to help your future performance, so you should aim to include this in your answer.

Experience of teaching (including outside medicine). Please identify the teaching methods used and include any teaching of junior postgraduate trainees, and any training in teaching.

Poor answer

I enjoy teaching having given general medical tutorials to fellow doctors during lunchtime teaching sessions. I have also taught clinical skills for 'Finals'. I have used a variety of different teaching formats such lectures and practical workshops. I seek formal feedback using written forms to improve my skills. Recognizing that training in teaching is essential, I have attended teaching courses. Outside of medicine, I have taught lifestyle drawing classes, teaching members of the public pencil and ink drawing. I find the variety of learner styles to be challenging meaning I need to adapt my teaching styles to everyone's differing needs.

This answer is too vague and may not convince the reader about the teaching performed. Name the lectures given and state which courses you attended and how they helped you. Also, it is helpful to show insight into why you seek feedback and how that helps your performance. This example could have used the non-medical section to demonstrate how the candidate can adapt their teaching style, for example by splitting the class into groups.

This question is actually very similar to the first but potentially allows you to be more generic. Don't fall into this trap. Short-listers like to see evidence (which they will want to see also at interview) and giving details helps them know you're not fibbing! Try and cram in as much of your teaching experience as possible, and ensure you describe your methods and use the appropriate buzzwords. As mentioned previously, it is important to mention the teacher training courses attended. Often application forms have another box or space to list courses attended, but the short-lister may have forgotten, or may be blinded to other parts of the form. Therefore gain your marks and emphasize your strengths. Go on the courses!

8 Audit and research

Elizabeth A Owen and Marc A Gladman

Introduction

Designers of the specialty training (ST) application process must have had a cruel sense of irony to bestow such disproportionate importance on the assessment of your knowledge of audit and research during the selection process for ST posts, given that it is arguably the most tedious of the topics encountered.

Unlike any other topic, there have been sections on *both* audit and research on ST application forms in *every* single specialty and in *every* single round of applications thus far, just as was the case previously with respect to Specialist Register (SpR) application forms.

There is no escaping this subject and if this hasn't convinced you to read this chapter, questions on these topics also constitute one-third of those asked at ST interviews (see Section C later in this book).

It is no exaggeration to say that there is no better way to jeopardize your chances of being appointed than by having a suboptimal grasp of the principles of audit and research and to lack examples to demonstrate your understanding of these topics.

The personal specification for ALL specialties states that applicants need to:

'Demonstrate an understanding of the importance of audit and research and the potential to contribute to development in medicine/ surgery/paediatrics, etc.' To be demonstrated on application form and at interview.

It is crucial to keep this statement in mind when preparing to tackle questions on the form.

Clinical audit

Thankfully, there are only four things that you need to know about clinical audit:

1. Definition
2. Aims
3. Steps involved
4. Skills acquired following participation.

We will discuss each of these in turn and then assimilate all the information to show you how to maximize your scores when presented with questions on the application form.

1. Definition: what is audit?

Actual definition:

'*Clinical audit aims to improve patient outcomes by improving professional practice and the general quality of services delivered. This is achieved through a continuous process where health-care professionals review patient care against agreed standards and make changes, where necessary, to meet those standards. The audit is then repeated to see if the changes have been made and the quality of patient care improved.*' Healthcare Commission, 2004.

Working definition of audit:

A process to compare *actual* clinical practice with an agreed *ideal* (gold standard), with a view to making changes if there is a discrepancy to improve patient care.

2. Aims: what is the relevance of audit?

Audit can be applied in different settings to evaluate structure (e.g. facilities, such as equipment/staffing level, etc.), process (e.g. activities such as investigations/treatment) or outcome (e.g. comparison with an ideal such as morbidity and mortality audits).

Q: *What is the purpose of clinical audit?*

A: The goals of audit can be to determine whether:

- what ought to be happening is happening – to identify weaknesses or failures
- current practice meets required standards – to identify good practice
- current practice follows published guidelines
- clinical practice is applying the knowledge that has been gained through research
- current evidence is being applied in a given situation.

Further aims are to:

- justify the use of resources and methods
- change clinical practice, where necessary, improving/ optimizing patient care or to improve the efficiency of a system/ department.

3. What are the steps involved in audit?

There are six steps involved in successfully completing an audit loop. The old terminology of an 'audit loop' has been superseded by referring to the process as an 'audit cycle', given that it may be necessary to go round more than once (essentially creating a spiral and not a loop!). We suggest using the **six Cs** to help you remember the steps involved.

The steps involved in audit: the six Cs

- Consider current clinical practice – observe what is going on
- Construct standards of care – using evidence-based guidelines/protocols
- Check (i.e. monitor) current practice against these standards
- Compare (quantitatively) current practice against the ideal gold standard
- Change instigation as appropriate
- Close the audit cycle

4. Skills acquired following participation in audit

This is the most common place where applicants drop points when answering questions on audit. You must demonstrate what you have learnt from your participation and reflect upon it.

Q: *What skills are gained from participation in audit?*

A: Demonstrate the following skills to the selectors to maximize your scores:

- Recognition of the importance in clinical governance
- Recognition of a problem or identification of an area of possible improvement – shows independent thinking and initiative
- Ability to perform literature searches and find best practice/gold standards – recognize good research
- Design of an investigation, setting of parameters – finding the best approach
- Data collection, cooperation with colleagues, working in a team
- Computer skills
- Statistical analysis, meaningful representation and interpretation of results
- Presentation of findings – public speaking, presentation skills
- Diplomacy and constructive criticism
- Innovation and problem-solving skills in suggesting and implementing changes
- Time and people management

Recognize any of these from personal specifications?

Practical approach to answering clinical audit questions

It is critical to demonstrate to the selectors that you fully appreciate the process and implications of clinical audit. More importantly, you must be able to communicate the skills that you have acquired from participating in an audit (i.e. 'give the selectors what they want') and reflect upon these new skills and their relevance to your training.

Do **NOT** merely regurgitate a definition of audit or use the allocated word count waffling on about the scenario/ background to your audit project. You will lose more than 75% of the available marks, no matter how impressive the project was!

For most questions on audit, we recommend using the SPAR approach to structure your response (see Chapter 5).

Q: How do I apply the SPAR technique when answering questions on audit?

A: Structure your response as follows:

[Situation/problem]

Briefly define the background to your project and define the gold standard that you used for comparison.

[Action]

Explain your *own* level of involvement, paying attention to covering the relevant steps of the audit loop (use the six Cs) and describing the skills that you acquired during each step. The majority of the marks are available here!

[Result/reflection]

Finish strongly by identifying a 'definite outcome'; explain how what you found changed practice. Don't forget to reflect on what you have learnt; this provides further opportunity to convey the new skills that you have acquired to the selectors!

Please enter evidence below to show that you have initiated, completed and presented an audit project. How is what you did relevant to ST?

Poor response

Appropriate treatment of UTI in A+E; Another Hospital 11/2006 *– I researched current UTI diagnostic and treatment guidelines, finding there was no hospital policy. With colleagues, we designed the assessment tool and collected a share of the data, which we analysed and jointly presented the findings at department teaching. In conjunction with the pharmacy department we constructed a guideline to include a common antibiotic protocol and most importantly a strategy for following results of MSU sent from A+E. This is now available on the intranet and due to be re-audited.*

This response is far too narrative. There is excessive use of 'we', which makes the reader question how much the candidate really contributed. Furthermore, there is no reflection on what the candidate has learnt or its application to their forthcoming ST. The applicant has mistakenly talked through the entire audit cycle with no reflection or insight into what was learnt. This means that marks available have been lost.

Excellent response

[Situation/problem]
Whilst working in the emergency department, I suspected that the British Thoracic Society (BTS) guidelines for the management of acute severe asthma were not being followed. Thus, I conducted a prospective audit of all cases presenting in a 2-month period.

[Actions]
Together with a colleague, I retrieved the guidelines, learning how to search the published literature in so doing. I designed a data collection tool, which helped me develop my IT skills, and distributed it within the

resuscitation room and to the triage nurse in the department. I met some resistance but was able to accomplish my aim with careful explanation of the purpose of the audit, improving my ability to negotiate and engage my colleagues. I sought help from the audit department in quantitatively comparing current practice with the national standards. I then presented the findings at our local grand round, which improved my confidence when speaking publicly and being diplomatic when fielding questions.

[Result/relevance/reflection]

The audit demonstrated that in 48 of 99 attendances, the BTS guidelines were not followed. Following suggestion, we produced a laminated copy of the guidelines in all areas of the emergency department. A repeat audit, completed 3 months later, revealed an improvement to 85% adherence. I will now feel more confident working autonomously and appraising published guidelines as a specialty trainee. Further, I have realized the importance of striving for the absolute best standards of care for my patients through the audit process and was gratified to be able to contribute on this occasion. .

This response demonstrates exactly the sort of level you should be aiming at when completing questions on the application form and will score highly. Such detail will only be possible with higher word limits (250 words), which are often allowed for such questions. The structured use of the SPAR technique provides a logical, easy-to-read flow to the description.

 Use the SPAR technique to describe a recent audit project.

Research

For the sake of simplicity, we will also only ask you to know the *same* four things about research.

1. Definition: what is research?

Actual definition:

> 'Research can be defined as the attempt to derive generalisable new knowledge by addressing clearly defined questions with systematic and rigorous methods.' Research Governance Framework for Health and Social Care 2003.

Working definition of research:

The quest for new knowledge that can be applied to clinical practice to improve the quality of patient care.

2. Aims: what is the relevance of research?

The purpose of research is to advance medical knowledge. However, the degree of interest is variable between doctors, with some being purely researchers, others purely clinical and others a combination of the two.

Q: Why should doctors be bothered with research?

A: Medical research is relevant as it:

- Advances medical knowledge

- Encourages curiosity and questioning of clinical practice

- Provides research-friendly clinicians who can collaborate more effectively with basic scientists

- Provides investigators with important generic skills (see below).

3. What are the steps involved in conducting a research study?

Essentially, research involves the formulation of a clinically pertinent question (the hypothesis) that is tested (investigated) using appropriately designed studies (experiment) in an attempt to answer the original question. We again suggest using the *same* six Cs that you used previously to help you remember the steps involved.

The steps involved in research: the six Cs

- Consider a clinically relevant question that needs answering – hypothesis formulation

- Compare this question with the published literature to ensure that the answer isn't already known – i.e. ensure originality

- Construct an appropriate experimental design to test the hypothesis and answer the question

- Check to see which is the best population of subjects (patients) to study

- Close the uncertainty by answering the original question

- Change clinical practice as appropriate by publishing your findings

4. Skills acquired following participation in research

Again, marks are commonly lost for failing to extract the learning points from being involved in research and the new skills that you have acquired. As usual, you must reflect on what you have done and learnt.

Q: What skills are gained from participation in research?

A: Demonstrate the following skills to the selectors to maximize your scores:

- An inquisitive nature in formulating clinically pertinent questions.

- Initiative and insight into identifying deficiencies in our current medical knowledge.

- Ability to perform literature searches and identify important studies.

- Appraisal and relevance of the published literature, enabling you to personally make decisions about whether or not you will incorporate the findings of other studies into your own clinical practice.

- Understanding of ethical and legal processes.

- Ability to plan and design a study, taking into account power and anticipating results.

- Practical lab skills.

- Teamworking and negotiation skills.

- Autonomy, personal drive and time management.

- Data collection, reproducibility, quality control.

- Statistical analysis.

- Self-appraisal, critical analysis and understanding and interpretation of results.

- Representation and presentation of findings, publishing work, presenting skills.

Practical approach to answering research questions

Exactly the same considerations apply when answering questions about research as for audit (see above). Again, we urge you to structure your answer using the SPAR technique and don't forget to give the selectors 'what they want' by demonstrating the skills that you have newly acquired having been involved in research.

Describe your understanding of the importance of medical research to a trainee doctor. You may use examples to illustrate your answer, either from your own experience or from publications if you have not had the opportunity to be involved in research.

Good response

Well-conducted research forms the cornerstone of evidence-based medicine which we strive to practise. The pursuit of new knowledge using systematic methods ensures medical advancement with a goal of achieving improvements in patient care and outcomes.

My research into factors affecting IVF success, specifically involved the identification of metabolites found in follicular fluid and influences on successful oocyte retrieval and fertilization.

Participation enabled me to develop an understanding of the ethics and practicalities of conducting research. Crucially, I was able to learn about study design under the supervision of the senior investigator. I was personally responsible for conducting the studies and collecting the data. I was able to develop skills in statistical analysis. I have learnt how to search the published literature and became conversant with the critical appraisal of other published studies. I also developed delicate experimental techniques that required a high degree of dexterity that should prove useful as a gynaecological surgeon in the future.

I was fortunate enough to be able to present my findings at a national scientific meeting and publish them in a peer-reviewed journal. Most importantly, it has stimulated me to be inquisitive in my clinical practice and to constantly consider whether such practice is based on evidence or tradition. Now that I can confidently appraise published research and determine its quality, I hope to incorporate the latest advances into clinical management of my patients.

 If you have undertaken or are undertaking a research project, please give details and indicate your level of involvement.

9 Clinical governance

Mark Portou

As with research and audit (see Chapter 8), your knowledge of clinical governance is likely to be tested not only within the application form but also during the interview. It is thus essential that you have a detailed understanding of this topic. For the purposes of this chapter, emphasis will be weighted towards answering questions encountered on the application form relating to clinical governance. However, you should also consult Section C of this book for examples of questions related to clinical governance that are encountered during the interview process.

Clinical governance is formally described as: '*a system through which NHS organizations are accountable for continuously improving the quality of their services and safeguarding high standards of care by creating an environment in which excellence in clinical care will flourish*'.

- The term 'clinical governance' was first coined in 1998 in the Department of Health publication: *A first class service: Quality in the new NHS*. Available at: http://www.dh.gov.uk/PublicationsAndStatistics/Publications/PublicationsPolicyAndGuidance/PublicationsPolicyAndGuidanceArticle/fs/en?CONTENT_ID=4006902&chk=j2Tt7C" \t "_blank".

Clinical governance is thus an NHS system for improving the standard of clinical care, through both detection, and correction of, poor performance, and the further improvement of successful practice. The implementation and structure of clinical governance was originally based around the 'Seven Pillars' of clinical governance, and these 'pillars' were held up by five 'foundation stones'. This model of describing 'pillars' is somewhat outdated now and has been replaced by a model of 'elements'.

A useful way of describing clinical governance is as an encompassing term for several '*elements*':

- Education and training
- Clinical audit
- Clinical effectiveness
- Research and development
- Openness
- Risk management

Use the acronym ERRORS to remember these elements:

Education and training

Risk management

Research and development

Openness

Reflection of practice (clinical audit)

Success (clinical effectiveness)

Elements such as risk management seek to identify potential systemic weaknesses in institutional practices and through the clinical governance processes, develop safeguards against these weaknesses. It is these potential flaws in any system, which when associated with human error, can lead to patient harm, failure or other adverse event.

The Department of Health White Paper '*An organisation with a memory*', published in 1998, explains the concepts of the 'person-centred approach' and 'system approach' to failure. The person-centred approach is the more traditional explanation for failures, using individual errors such as 'inattention, forgetfulness and carelessness' to explain error. This approach was favourable to organizations as it concentrates on individuals, predisposing to disciplinary proceedings and 'blaming, naming and shaming'.

However, the system approach recognizes that error and failure are often due to a combination of factors, and that failures are inevitable. Further to this it understands that human error is unavoidable, but concentrates on the organizational issues and contexts that allowed the human mistake to occur, or that prevented the error from being identified and corrected. The system approach acknowledges that even the best people make mistakes, and that these mistakes often recur. The human error aspect occurs in two ways, through 'active failures' and 'latent conditions'.

Active failures describe the 'slips, lapses, mistakes and procedural violations' that occur leading to an incident; this describes the human error element. Latent conditions are more complicated, and describe procedures, practices and policies, which alone do not lead to critical incidents, but when combined with other factors have the potential to lead to patient harm.

 What do you understand by the term clinical governance?

This question is an obvious one and should be approached in terms of the official definition provided above. You should also demonstrate an *understanding* by mentioning the pillars, and better still, the elements of clinical governance.

Give evidence of your participation in the clinical governance process
or
Describe your experience of clinical governance

As an F2 in a regional endocrine surgical unit, I witnessed a critical incident involving a preoperative patient due to undergo a nephrectomy for a renal cell carcinoma. He had arrived late onto the ward the evening before surgery, and thus was clerked, site marked and consented by the cross covering general surgical SHO. Unfortunately the wrong side had been marked and consented for, and this mistake was only noticed seconds before anaesthesia was induced. Following this near miss, I undertook an audit into the pre op marking and consenting practice of this unit, and completed a route-cause analysis of this incident. My findings highlighted many latent errors in the system, such as lack of electronic viewers for CD-based patient radiology, and over reliance on out-of-hours cross covering individuals not present in theatre the next day. My findings and recommendations were presented at the department audit meeting.

Answering these questions will require the candidate to have an active knowledge of the elements of clinical governance (remember ERRORS). The simplest and most obvious way of answering this question is to describe an example of one of the elements. e.g. clinical audit (see Chapter 8) or 'risk management' or 'education and training', etc.

Where have you seen clinical governance in action?

In order to reduce the risk of patient harm occurring through inappropriate surgery, my current hospital trust has introduced the concept of a 'time out' system prior to commencing the operation. This involves the operating surgeon cross checking the patient bracelet details with the consent form in order to reduce the incidences of adverse events.

This is a more difficult question to answer, and requires knowledge of specific outcomes as a result of the now 10-year-old concept of clinical governance. Look around your individual hospital trust for such outcomes. To stimulate this thought process, nationally implemented outcomes include:

- National Patient Safety Agency (NPSA) hand-washing campaign
- Nationally standardized operating theatre checklists
- Complaints procedures
- IR1 Incident forms.

10 Professional integrity

Kamaldeep Manak, Megan Crofts and Marc A Gladman

- Professionalism: *professional character, spirit, or methods*
- Integrity: *adherence to moral and ethical principles; soundness of moral character; honesty*
- Professional integrity: *ability to do the right thing when faced with a situation that would be easier to ignore*

Probity and professional integrity are highlighted as key features of the General Medical Council's *Good Medical Practice* guidelines. Consequently, it is not surprising that questions on this topic are commonly encountered within the specialty training application process.

Provide a specific example of a work situation where professional integrity was required on your part. What approach did you take and how did your actions demonstrate integrity?

Q: How should I break down this question when planning my response?

A: Using the **SPAR** technique, break this question down into its three key components:

- **Situation/problem:** identify a *specific* example of a *work* situation that demonstrates professional integrity
- **Actions:** Explain the approach you took
- **Reflection:** Explain how your actions display professional integrity

1. Identify a specific example of a work situation that demonstrates professional integrity

As discussed in Chapter 5, the example you chose here should meet the PRO criteria and preferably should incorporate one of your 'big guns' if at all possible, although it is often difficult to achieve this with questions such as this. You may have to save your big gun for another question and instead search for the most original example with which to impress the selectors this question.

Suitable examples that may demonstrate professional integrity include:

- Difficult or failing colleagues or seniors with the potential to impact on patient care
- Situations where you acknowledged and worked within your limitations
- Patient confidentiality issues, e.g. consent
- Communication problems
- Accidental non-fatal medical errors

Make sure that you do NOT:

- **Define an action as demonstrating 'professional integrity' when it doesn't**
- **Make yourself look more professional than a colleague**
- **Describe dealing with complex situations on your own**
- **Ignore the feelings of the patient/person concerned**

2. Explain the approach that you took

As explained in Chapter 5, this section of your response is where most of the marks will be awarded and thus you should allocate the most significant proportion of the word count to explaining *what you did*. Depending on the example you chose, you will need to demonstrate certain actions, as shown in the following example.

If you choose to describe an accidental non-fatal medical error, use the acronym MISTAKE to help you highlight the salient points in your response:

- **Make good the situation to prevent patient harm**
- **Immediate recognition/action**
- **Senior involvement (Specialist Registrar/consultant)**
- **Transparent**
- **Apology (if appropriate)**
- **Kritical incident reporting**
- **Every possible step possible was taken to correct the mistake**

3. Explain how your actions display professional integrity

Having described what actions you took, you need to finish your response with a 'strong concluding statement' that describes:

- The outcome
- Reflection of what you have learnt as a consequence of the incident.

Ensure that you convey to the person marking the response that you have learnt from and reflected on the incident and will not make a similar mistake in the future. Better still, explain how the episode can be avoided by others in the future.

- **All too often, applicants are so relieved at finishing the descriptive part of the response that they fail to make a concluding statement relating to the outcome of the scenario and what has been learnt from it.**
- **This will result in you dropping potential marks.**
- **Aim to avoid weak endings that 'tail off' and aim for a strong positive statement of reflection so that you finish the response on a 'high'.**

Provide a specific example of a work situation where professional integrity was required on your part. What approach did you take and how did your actions demonstrate integrity?

Worked example

[Situation/problem]

Whilst working in a busy, overbooked outpatient clinic, I inadvertently prescribed bowel preparation for a patient that I'd booked to undergo a gastroscopy, mixing her up with the previous patient I saw who needed to undergo a colonoscopy.

[Action]

*Whilst dictating my clinic letters, I realized what had happened (**immediate recognition**). I immediately informed my consultant (**seniors involved**) and reviewed the patient's records to retrieve her contact details (**every step possible taken**). I contacted her the same afternoon (**make good the situation**) and apologized (**apology**) that I had prescribed the bowel preparation in error. I confirmed that it was not necessary for her gastroscopy and that she should not take it. On the advice of my boss, I completed a critical incident form (**critical incident reporting**).*

[Result/reflection]

Subsequently, I have paid closer attention to my levels of tiredness, particularly when in busy clinical situations. I now meticulously check all investigations and prescriptions and ensure that I finish one task before moving on to the next. I have realized that every patient encounter can result in a bad outcome if adequate attention is not devoted to the task in hand.

Using an example from your experience to date, demonstrate how you have learnt from a potentially serious mistake/error and how your practice has changed as a result.

Poor response

During a geriatric attachment, a patient with dementia was commenced on aspirin for a newly diagnosed atrial fibrillation on a busy Consultant ward round. However, her old notes documented an unconfirmed allergy to aspirin. The pharmacist alerted me of this error. I approached the nurse who administrated the drug and demanding how she could make an error. I tried to confirm this allergic with the patient who was unhelpful due to the dementia. I then informed my Registrar who was angry and promptly assessed this patient. He discontinued the aspirin, asked the nurses to increase observations and completed an incident report.

In this answer, the candidate fails to embrace the importance of patient safety or take responsibility for the situation. Instead the candidate describes the actions of the registrar, blames the nursing staff and lacks empathy for the patient. The candidate does not reflect or seem to learn from this error. This example is also poorly written with grammatical errors. This demonstrates the importance of simple measures such as spell check as well as proofreading prior to submission. In summary, although this is a reasonable choice of example, the applicant fails to demonstrate an appreciation of the principles of probity.

Average response

During a geriatric attachment, a patient with dementia was commenced on aspirin for a newly diagnosed atrial fibrillation on a busy Consultant ward round. However, her old notes documented an unconfirmed allergy to aspirin. The pharmacist alerted me to this error. I promptly assessed this patient who could not confirm the allergy and did not exhibit any signs of an allergic response. I stopped aspirin, asked the nurses to increase observations and alerted my Registrar. The patient remained well however an incident report was completed. This incident has reinforced my safe clinical practice by checking allergy wristbands, obtaining a thorough drug allergy history, documenting allergic responses and collating information for those unable to communicate.

In this response, the applicant acted responsibly and made adequate efforts to maintain patient safety in a constructive and non-judgemental manner. The use of clinical incident reporting highlights an awareness of the importance of clinical risk management. However, this answer may be improved by elaborating upon the reflection. For example, involving the family to confirm the allergy and explaining the situation. In addition, it would also be prudent to discuss this with the prescribing doctor and consultant.

Good response

During a geriatric Consultant ward round, a patient with dementia was commenced on aspirin for newly diagnosed atrial fibrillation. However, an allergy to aspirin was documented in her old notes. The pharmacist alerted me to this error. I promptly assessed this patient who could not confirm the allergy and did not exhibit any signs of an allergic response. I discontinued aspirin and asked the nurses to increase observations. I informed the Registrar who reviewed the patient, agreed she was stable and commenced slow intravenous fluids. I informed the on call team SHO of this patient and attempted to validate this allergy with the patient's GP and next of kin. I informed the Consultant of this error and completed an incident report in a transparent and constructive manner. I remained calm, professional and honest throughout this stressful situation. This incident has reinforced my safe clinical practice by checking allergy wristbands, obtaining a thorough drug history, documenting allergic responses and collating information for those unable to communicate.

Describe an incident that demonstrates your professionalism and/or integrity. Highlight your actions and the consequences.

This question is very similar to the first but more vague. Although the question does not ask you to reflect, it is crucial that you add at least a sentence on what you have learnt or may have changed. This highlights that you have learnt from the error and enhanced your personal and professional development.

Poor response

During a shift in the Minors department in <u>A+E</u>, I saw a patient who had slipped over in her kitchen and was now complaining of left <u>ankel</u> pain. I ordered an x-ray. I didn't see any abnormalities in it and sent the patient home. When <u>I was discussed</u> the case at the end of the shift, my senior realized I had missed a fracture. He made me call the patient and get her to return to the department for a plaster of <u>paris.</u> <u>I now have to</u> discuss all radiographs with my seniors and had to go on an <u>xray</u> course.

The above example demonstrates several of the 'what not to do' points. The basic errors of spelling and the grammar are underlined and are simple to correct; use a spell check and get other people to read it. Whatever examples you choose to use, showing that you take responsibility for your actions and decisions is important, as well as showing how you've learnt from the error or the specific experience and how it has changed your practice in the long term.

Good response

I was working in the minors department of Accident and Emergency, when a mobile patient presented complaining of left ankle pain, having slipped in her kitchen. The patient underwent an x-ray of her ankle, but I failed to identify the hairline fracture of her distal fibula. I discharged the patient with analgesia and arranged follow-up if the pain should continue. I reviewed the x-ray later on in the shift with a senior, and my error was identified. Having notified the Consultant, I then endeavoured to contact the patient and organized for her to return to the department, where a full explanation and apology was given, and the patient fully treated. I completed an incident form, and discussed the case fully with the Consultant afterwards, and have since attended a Radiology course.

The applicant identifies an error, and swiftly takes responsibility in correcting it, whilst seeking advice and involving all the necessary senior parties. The applicant also shows that they have reflected fully on how the error occurred, and identified weaknesses in their knowledge, and took swift action to rectify this by taking a course. In reading this answer, we get the impression that we can trust this person, and depend on them to act with integrity and honesty.

Describe an incident that demonstrates your professionalism and/or integrity. Highlight your actions and the consequences.

You admit a previously independent and well 80-year-old woman for i.v. antibiotics having diagnosed her with a lower lobe pneumonia. Your registrar tells you to withhold all treatment, 'she's 80 years old and it would be a waste of resources to treat someone so old'. Is your registrar right? How would you deal with this situation? Who else would you involve?

11 The patient as the central focus of care

Anna Barrow

The first principle of Good Medical Practice is to ensure that the care of your patients is your first concern. It is your duty to protect and promote the health of the patient, to treat patients as individuals, respecting their dignity and their right to confidentiality, and to work in partnership with your patients. The doctor–patient relationship has changed in recent years, from a doctor-led, didactic model to a partnership of care whereby the patient is the main focus and where the doctor and patient act together to decide on the best management plan.

Changes in the NHS have aimed to achieve a more patient-friendly model of care and are being led through patient focus and public involvement alongside governance and assessment of standards. Patient focus means maintaining good communication with patients as individuals and as communities and groups. Public interaction ensures that services are targeted at individual and community specific needs. This keeps patients involved in and updated on the services available to them.

Patient focus involves four key components:

- Improving services and communication with the users of services, including feedback
- Dissemination of information
- Encouragement of patient involvement
- Responsiveness to issues identified

Do not get stuck in describing the now out-dated 'departmental' or specialty-based system of care. Contemporary patient care involves a more integrated service with use of 'clinical pathways' to provide recognized standards for care.

Give an example of something you did recently that had a positive effect on a patient's care.

Poor response

In my time as a house officer, I was involved in caring for an elderly woman who had been in hospital for many weeks on the elderly medicine ward and was getting very lonely. She was seen every morning on the ward rounds and was just awaiting placement in a longer stay hospital as she was failing to cope at home. As she rarely needed any investigations, I had not had much interaction with her. I was asked to repeat one of her blood tests and when I went to see her she asked me why she was still in hospital as no one had told her why she could not go home. She was concerned that she might have a terminal diagnosis which no one was telling her about. I sat down with her and explained why she was still in hospital and the plans for her future care and she was very relieved.

This poor response takes too long setting the scene and pays little attention to how the applicant's actions had a positive effect on the patient. Further explanation about why the action improved the patient's care is needed, followed by reflection about how this could be used to improve other patients' care. The answer should provide an opportunity for you to show how you have gone over and above your duty to help a patient and what you have learnt from the experience that you can take forward.

Better response

> *Whilst working as an SHO in a sexual health clinic, I saw a 16-year-old girl. She was initially nervous and it was difficult to take her history. However, I was non-judgemental and I tried to put her at ease. I reassured her that the consultation was fully confidential. She had presented as she was concerned that she might have contracted a sexually transmitted infection. I ascertained that she was using no contraception and on further questioning, this was due to incorrect health-care beliefs. I counselled her regarding contraception, safe sex and referred her to the family planning nurse. She left the clinic with a better understanding of sexual health and an understanding of how to take responsibility for her own health. I was able to learn that one may have to be opportunistic with health-care promotion issues, identifying problems and educating patients during the consultation.*

This answer demonstrates how the candidate's actions have a positive impact on the patient's care both short and long term. The answer highlights the use of education in health-care promotion and also discusses key concepts such as changing health-care beliefs and involvement of other health-care professionals to provide a holistic approach to patient care. Marks will be awarded for demonstrating not only how you have improved a situation but also for recognizing how this was achieved so that it can be used in the future.

Give an example of how good communication made a difference to patient care.

Poor response

> *As a medical student I took part in a communication skills course which taught me the basics of breaking bad news. As a junior doctor I attended a communication skills lecture and workshop on communication with patients. I always try to keep my patients up to date with their progress and try to build a good rapport.*

This answer should contain two main parts: (i) demonstration of how your communication skills stand out and (ii) how something you did affected patient care followed by consideration of why it made a difference. The above answer fails to make the candidate stand out. Most medical students have completed a communication skills course and keeping your patient informed is part of *standard* good practice. The answer fails to identify a factor in the patient's care that made a difference and how this was achieved through good communication. The use of reflection, evidence of going beyond your job remit and showing your skills not only in communication with the patient but also with other team members in terms of note keeping and verbal communication will secure marks for such questions.

Better response

Whilst working in Emergency Medicine, I saw a patient who spoke no English. At initial assessment, I was concerned that she was septic and began initiating resuscitation and summoned senior help. I ascertained that neither she nor her husband spoke much English. Since it was out of hours, I called 'language line' to get a clear history from her husband whilst arranging for an advocate. Unfortunately, her condition deteriorated rapidly and I moved her to resus area of the department and contacted the ITU registrar. I ensured that I documented the history clearly and arranged for close follow up. In this case I endeavoured to communicate as best I could with the patient and her family despite language barriers. I also communicated the urgency of this case and the need to escalate and expedite her care with the rest of my team. On reflection, I felt I had made a difference ensuring that her care was expedited and also by trying to overcome language barriers which might have made it difficult to get important details relating to her care as well as making the patient and her family more aware of the situation and how we were managing her.

This answer highlights difficulties encountered in trying to communicate with a patient and how they were overcome. The doctor reflects on why the situation went well and what was learnt from it. It describes the involvement of other members of the team to assist (escalation) and demonstrates a safe approach with consideration for the patient and her family at the same time as managing the medical side of things. The answer also draws reference to good written communication and accurate note keeping as well as referrals and verbal communications.

 What would you do if a patient disagreed with your treatment approach?

Poor response

If a patient disagreed with my treatment approach, I would try to persuade them to cooperate with treatment and explain that it was for their own good. I would ask them why they did not want to take the medication prescribed and explain that it was the best thing to give them. If the patient still disagreed then I would ask a senior to help and try to resolve the problem. I would remember the patient's right to a second opinion.

This answer fails to take account of the patient being the focus of care. It ignores the concept of a partnership of care between doctor and patient, whereby a mutual understanding and management plan is reached. While the doctor rightly explained that the treatment was for the good of the patient, he/she did not discuss alternative options or take into account the reasons why the patient did not agree. It is possible that the patient was unable to tolerate a medication, perhaps it did not suit their lifestyle, perhaps they were unable to attend appointments for treatments when needed, or perhaps they had read something worrying about a particular treatment. Eliciting the patient's agenda helps to identify the true problem. Discussions about alternatives can then take place to reach a compromise and regain the patient's trust and confidence in the doctor.

Better answer

As an SHO in GUM clinic, I saw a patient with HIV who was non-compliant with her medications. I tried to build a rapport with the patient and establish a no-blame attitude in ascertaining her reasons for not taking her medications. It turned out that she was now living in shared-accommodation and was unable to keep her medications in the fridge in case her flatmates found them. It was difficult for her to follow a strict dosing regime due to her work and study commitments and she had also suffered some side effects. She was dubious about the need for antiretrovirals since she felt well. We discussed the risks of not taking her medications correctly which she had not fully understood. I involved my consultant and a nurse specialist to discuss alternative treatment options and a change in her drug regimen to allow her more flexibility was proposed. We gave her information about sources of support. Two weeks later she returned and her blood tests showed that the drugs were working well. I realised on reflection how important it is to listen to a patient fully and to ascertain their agendas when discussing management options.

This answer remembers that the patient is the centre of focus and takes into account the patient's reasons for non-compliance or disagreement. It also demonstrates a degree of empathy with the patient and involvement of other sources of help from health-care professionals and dissemination of information in a way the patient can understand, ensuring education to change her health beliefs and behaviours. Importantly, it also reflects upon the importance of empathizing and listening to patients in order to develop a trusting doctor–patient relationship.

12 Teamwork and leadership skills

Shalini Kawar and Anna Barrow

As a doctor, the ability to work effectively alongside others is crucial, as well as a more directive, leadership role in other aspects of work. Debate exists as to whether teamwork and leadership skills relate to inherent personal qualities possessed by individuals of a particular personality type, or whether they are skills that can be learnt, practised and developed. In any case they are two areas commonly assessed during the specialty training (ST) application process. To demonstrate that you possess these skills when answering questions on the application form and at interview effectively will require an understanding of what constitutes a successful team player and leader.

Teamwork

> A team is defined as a group of people with complementary skills, who are committed to a common purpose, performance goals, and an approach for which they are mutually accountable.

Good teamwork ensures that goals are achieved efficiently and successfully.

Formation of an effective team can be a protracted process, which can be divided into discrete stages:

1. FORMING: early on people tend to be guarded, self-aware, polite.
2. STORMING: controlled conflict may follow initial confusion and there may be difficulty agreeing methods or goals.
3. NORMING: as time progresses, the team becomes more organized and clear roles and feedback processes are established.

Doctors are a key part of the multidisciplinary team (MDT). It is important that all members of the team have clearly defined roles recognized by all. Members must be appreciative of the skill mix available and aware of overlap and boundaries of individual roles. One clear leader or facilitator is usually agreed, but confusion over authority can arise in an MDT where hierarchical relationships are somewhat skewed by the presence of different professionals, grades, ages and experience. MDTs are also affected by rapid staff turnover: shift systems mean that different staff may be covering each role at different times, people move on to different departments, and various emergencies and urgencies may mean that people are missing at various times.

In recent ST applications, the person specifications identified teamwork as a desirable characteristic, as 'the capacity to work cooperatively with others and work effectively in an MDT'. This characteristic is commonly assessed on the application form and at interview. To be able to answer such questions effectively, it is important to know the characteristics of *both* the team and individual teamworkers.

Characteristics of a successful teamworker

- Treats others with respect
- Is willing to help
- Is flexible and open to taking on ideas that may differ from their own
- Demonstrates good communication skills as well as good listening skills
- Is reliable
- Is responsible for their own contribution within the team

Characteristics of teamwork

- The goals should be discussed and agreed by all members of the team

- There must be effective communication skills that ensure free flow of information between team members

- The relationship between members of the team should be supportive and trusting

- If disagreement should arise, this should be orientated around the goal, and not directed towards individuals

- The atmosphere should be non-threatening and non-competitive

- Team roles should be defined clearly

Typical teamwork questions from recent ST application forms include:

- *What makes a good team?*

- *What are the attributes of a good team player?*

- *Do you work better as part of a team or on your own?*

- *Give us a recent example of a time where you worked as a member of an MDT.*

- *Give an example of how you have solved a complex problem through teamwork. What did you learn from this experience?*

- *Explain a time when you successfully worked within a team.*

- *Tell us about a less successful team. What went wrong?*

- *Who are the most important people within a team?*

- *What are the advantages and disadvantages of a doctor working as part of a team?*

- *Please describe any experience of working closely with other people. You may give examples of both inside and outside medicine.*

Approach to questions on teamwork

Refer to Chapter 5 for a reminder of the generic approach to questions. Specifically, for questions on teamwork, you should aim to demonstrate that you are aware of the qualities of a successful teamworker. The questions may also ask you to demonstrate, with examples, situations where you have displayed such skills or identified them in others. These questions may relate to your medical training so far, or may be broader and ask for examples from other areas of your life, such as sporting activities.

When answering these questions, the SPAR framework can be used, highlighting its applicability to all questions on the application form.

Use of SPAR when answering teamwork questions

If asked to describe a situation where you worked successfully as part of a team, your question should be structured as follows:

- S: What team you were part of; where this team was based

- P: What the goals of the team were; what your own role was

- A: How you went about achieving this goal, both personally and collectively as a group

- R: What the end result was, and how this impacted on others; what you have learnt from this experience and how this is relevant to specialist training

Q: How should I approach questions on teamwork?

A: Use a structured approach:

- Think of a situation where you have worked as part of a team

- Review the skills assessed using the personal specification

- Remind yourself of the qualities of a successful team/team player as outlined above

- Reflect on what you have learnt about teamwork

Suitable examples when answering questions on teamwork:

1. Sporting events

2. Public performances, e.g. concerts

3. Research projects

4. Charity fundraising

5. Medical school-related events

6. Realized business ideas

7. Expeditions

8. Jobs

It is easy to answer a teamwork question by using the words 'team', 'teamworker' and 'teamworking' as many times as possible but at the same time failing to clearly define your role within that team.

Leadership skills

Working in the health-care profession, you will have to adapt to many different situations. Simply being a good team player may not be enough to succeed in the working environment, nor during job applications or interviews. One day you may take on a passive role within a team, for example writing notes during a ward round, but then you may have to take the lead with junior colleagues, such as during teaching sessions. Leadership skills, therefore, are as important as teamworking skills.

To effectively answer questions examining your leadership skills you need to understand about different leadership styles and the qualities of a good leader so that you can communicate this information to the selectors.

Leadership styles

Autocratic

This is the classic approach, whereby the leader retains as much power over decision making as possible. Other members are expected to obey orders and are not allowed to have much input. This method can be used successfully in situations where members are new and untrained, and are not aware of how things should be done. This type of leadership can also be useful if there is limited time during which a task needs to be performed. The downside of this, however, may be low team morale, absenteeism, or a fearful and resentful working environment.

Bureaucratic

This form of leadership is where tasks are performed in accordance with policy and protocols. This is useful when routine tasks are performed repeatedly, or in situations where safety is a major concern. However, it can result in the formation of habits that are hard to deviate from. Also, team members may do only what is expected of them, as they are not encouraged to initiate new ideas or approaches.

Democratic

This is where team members are encouraged to be involved in decision making. This keeps them informed and shares the responsibilities between individuals. However, if there are many team members, this approach may not be practical. It may be more efficient for the leader to make the decisions, and saves the leader from feeling that his or her role is being threatened.

Laissez-faire or 'hands off'

Here, the leader provides little or no direction, and all members of the team are given as much freedom as possible. The individuals of the team are encouraged to set goals, make decisions and resolve problems on their own. This is particularly useful if everyone is at a similar level of skill and experience. Therefore, if there are less experienced, more junior members of the team, this will not be successful.

The style of leadership adopted will depend on factors such as:

- the leader's background (e.g. personality, experience, ethics and values);
- the attributes of the 'followers' (e.g. personalities, background and experience); and
- the nature of the organization (e.g. values, philosophy and concerns, etc.).

Q: What are the qualities of a good leader?

A: The following tend to make an individual a good leader:

- Has clear objectives of the task in hand and is able to communicate and delegate these to the team

- Sets an example to the rest of the group

- Is familiar with members of the team and knows how to motivate them

- Has effective communication and listening skills

- Is decisive

- Is open to suggestions from other team members, and understands the need for change

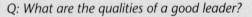

Typical questions about leadership on recent ST application forms include:

- *What are the qualities of a good/bad leader?*

- *What does 'leading by example' mean to you?*

- *What leadership skills have you acquired during your training?*

- *How would you motivate others?*

- *Tell us about a situation where you showed leadership.*

- *Describe any management/leadership roles you have been involved with at work.*

Describe a situation where you showed leadership. (150 words)

Poor response

I know what makes a good leader and by watching others and having the chance to practice these skills, I have successfully taken on several leadership roles. At work I always take a lead whenever possible. I have run cardiac arrests and shown a leadership role during ward rounds when I delegate jobs to nurses and juniors. I always volunteer to teach junior colleagues and helped arrange a teaching programme for them in preparation for their final exams. Their feedback was very positive and they all passed, which indicates the success of these sessions. Although I believe I possess effective leadership skills, I hope to develop these further during the course of my future jobs.

In this response the applicant merely informs us that he/she possesses leadership skills, rather than demonstrating the application of such skills using a well-illustrated example. This response would score badly.

Better response

During my FY2 year, I set up a journal club for my colleagues. Some of my fellow FY doctors were keen to involve themselves in the organizational side of things. I looked at their individual skills and preference and delegated roles and responsibilities accordingly. As popularity grew, so did my role in maintaining an organized and stimulating group. I held regular meetings to maintain effective communication within the team to ensure an efficient working environment. Although I took overall leadership, I welcomed suggestions from other members in order to provide the best educational benefit to all.

From regular feedback, I was pleased to learn others found me approachable and supportive.

Upon leaving the hospital, I handed over responsibility to a junior doctor who was keen to take over. Speaking to a colleague who still works there, the group is still being held and maintains its popularity.

This is a relatively simple scenario, but covers the leadership skills in a demonstrable way. The candidate here would come across as someone who clearly knows the qualities of a successful leader, and has included several key elements, for example, 'approachable', 'supportive', 'regular communication with the team', 'delegate roles depending on skill mix'. All of these help form a good answer.

Please describe any experience of working closely with other people. You may give examples of both inside and outside medicine.

What leadership skills have you acquired during your training?

13 Clinical prioritization and time management

Beverley Almeida

A vital skill for a doctor is knowing how to prioritize work; an imperative part of our job is how to arrange and deal with jobs in order of importance. It is an essential skill to have so that you can make the best use of your time and efforts, thus ensuring the best care for your patients and their management. In our careers as doctors, where time is limited but demands seem to be unlimited, it helps to allocate your time where it is most needed, allowing less important tasks to be attended to later. In essence, questions on this topic within the application form are evaluating your ability to prioritize your workload and manage your time effectively.

The key to answering questions on this topic is to convey that:

- you are a safe doctor who doesn't do things that put your patients at risk

- you are willing to ask for help if you feel out of your depth

- you would work as a team and share jobs with your fellow doctors

Describe a specific example from your experience in this specialty of a time when you had to cope with the pressure of various stressful clinical situations at the same time. What strategies did you adopt to complete all the tasks asked of you?

Let's assume that you had to prioritize the following three situations to answer this question:

1. A patient's cannula has tissued.
2. A relative is waiting to speak to you, he does not sound happy.
3. A patient on a morphine PCA has just received a bolus 10 times the prescribed dose.

Think about this as though you might if you were given these choices in real life. Clearly, scenario 3 is the most urgent, the patient could be in imminent danger; followed by scenario 2 as an unhappy person could turn into an angry person and you have a potential for averting a confrontational encounter if you can deal with it promptly. Whether scenario 1 should be more important than scenario 2 depends on having further details. So, you do not have much room in the white space of 150 words to deal with this, but it is possible if you follow the SPAR technique.

Poor response

There were 3 cases I had: a patient whose cannula had tissued, a relative who wanted an update and a patient on a morphine PCA who received a dangerous bolus. I made an immediate decision to deal with the new cannula first. This was a quick and straightforward job, so I got this out of the way and then headed over to the patient with the morphine bolus. When I attended I stopped any further morphine being administered, asked the nurses to do some observations and assessed the patient for any adverse signs. Once stabilized I left instructions with the nurses to call me, only if the patient was deteriorating. I then went and sorted out the irate relative. I considered apologising for the delay as he felt he had been kept waiting, but didn't and then tried to set about allaying his concerns and listening to him. (148 words)

Q: What makes this a poor response?

A: This is a poor response as:

- There is no clear reasoning here, all decisions seem to be made on a whim.

- All the work was done by one person; there is not even any communication with the rest of the team. You are allowed to share jobs and work as a team!

- Treatment only occured once you were in front of the actual patient, thus delaying their care and there is no escalation of the fact that there is a sick patient on the ward.

- Further care is dumped onto the nurses, when in reality there are times when the same patient needs to be repeatedly reviewed by the same doctor, even if they have stabilized.

- It is always a good idea to say you're sorry. Sorry is not an admission of guilt and shows that you are an empathetic person. Many complaints are due to the fact that the only word people wanted the doctor to say was sorry and they never heard it.

- Overall the language is too informal. It just doesn't instil the reader with confidence that you are a good doctor.

Better response

There were 3 cases I had to deal with: a patient whose cannula had tissued, a relative who wanted an update and a patient on a morphine PCA who had received a dangerous bolus. I first obtained more information, I checked why the patient needed a cannula and what the relative wanted to discuss. I obtained the observations of the final patient as well as verbally asking to stop any further administration. Recognizing my limitations, I contacted the other team members and delegated the cannulation to the FY1, asked the nurse to initially speak to the relative and the SpR to also speak to the relative later. I then attended to the patient with the excess morphine and assessed for hypotension, tachycardia and pinpoint pupils. I administered Naloxone, stabilized them and alerted my consultant and the patient of the mistake. I then checked with my colleagues if they needed any help. (150 words)

Q: What makes this a good response?

A: This is a good response as it demonstrates that:

- Further details are gained before you make any firm decisions
- Jobs are delegated and shared among the team – junior, senior and nursing
- Assistance is sought
- Treatment is initialized even before arriving at the patient's bedside
- The patient in danger is immediately recognized
- Knowledge about clinical incident reporting and risk management is demonstrated, as well as the signs to look for in a morphine overdose

Describe a situation where you had to respond quickly to unexpected and stressful circumstances at work. What did you do to achieve an acceptable outcome in this situation?

Example answer

As the only SpR on night duty at a tertiary neonatal unit, there was a sick term infant at a peripheral hospital who needed to be retrieved. I needed extra help, so contacted the consultant on call to make sure the unit had senior cover whilst the child was transported to us. I enlisted my SHO to check how busy labour ward was and asked the senior midwife to inform us as soon as there may be any potential preterm deliveries. As a nurse practitioner was already at work, I also asked her to cover any urgent jobs. My consultant arrived to take over responsibility of the unit and I travelled to the peripheral hospital with one of the senior nurses. The baby was retrieved successfully and safely, while in my absence the SHO had felt well supported by the senior members I had left at the unit. (149 words)

Describe a time when you had a particularly difficult day at work. What strategies did you use to cope with this situation both during and after this time and how effective were they?

Example answer

I was working on nights in A&E with only myself and a locum covering the department. I was relatively inexperienced and we were struggling with the workload. I remained calm and informed the Sister in Charge and the Night Matron of the situation and suggested that I speak to the medical and surgical teams on call to directly admit several of the patients, with their cooperation. The Night Matron had worked in a minor injuries unit and so was able to see some of the patients, freeing me up to see the more urgent cases. By taking regular breaks and employing a methodical approach I was able to take control of the situation and ensure that we worked well as a team. The following morning I debriefed with a senior colleague and then went cycling, allowing me to realise that a potentially stressful situation had become a valuable learning experience. (150 words)

The above examples prioritize communication with colleagues in order to complete the tasks in an organized and professional fashion. The first example is more specific about patient safety, which should be the first consideration and should be specifically mentioned in these scenarios.

- Put patient safety first
- Show good communication with colleagues
- Act professionally, no glory and no blame
- Reflect

14 Coping under pressure

Jasdeep Gill and Sukhjinder Nijjer

Introduction

Pressure is intrinsic within the jobs and lives of all doctors. The ability to understand and cope under pressure is an essential quality for doctors; however, this is a skill that can take years to hone. Being placed under pressure can be a positive thing but poor mechanisms to cope under pressure can leave some doctors feeling physically and emotionally exhausted. You will notice that each job specification states coping with pressure as an *essential* criterion. Therefore, being able to cope with pressure and demonstrate this on your specialty training (ST) application form is a critical skill that will serve you and your future patients.

This chapter will discuss the importance of identifying stressors, how to cope with pressure and how to tackle these questions using worked examples. You may have already developed a number of coping mechanisms subconsciously, some of which will be good but others less so. We will discuss ideal coping mechanisms that you can use, not only on a daily basis, but to also help stimulate ideas for your application form answers.

Identifying stressors

To cope with stress successfully it is important that you are aware of the pressure(s) and identify the root cause. Look critically at your day-to-day tasks and the approach you use to solve problems. During your training so far, your posts will have differed in intensity and the level of stress you faced will have varied. Consider each post and identify what made each one difficult or easy. What factors contribute to your stress on a day-to-day level? Remember that the stressors in your life are likely to be multifactorial, so divide them broadly into categories, such as work and personal stressors, and then subdivide them from there.

Examples of 'stressors' experienced by doctors include:

Work-related

- Unwell patients
- Lack of experience or skills
- Lack of time to perform tasks
- Unhelpful management or administration
- Lack of control over your environment and the demands placed upon you
- Rota difficulties
- Lack of resources
- Lack of teamwork and team structure
- Communication difficulties with patients or staff members
- Seeking perfection with high self-expectations
- Feeling it is you against the 'system'
- NHS and hospital politics

Personal factors

- Insufficient leisure time
- Financial worries
- Family and social commitments
- Living arrangements
- Child-care issues
- Travelling issues

Suggested ways of coping under pressure

- Recognize stress, pressures and fatigue early
- Find time for regular relaxation, sleeping properly
- Take breaks
- Monitor your state of mind; become aware of stress indicators
- Manage your time by being more organized and prioritizing
- Be flexible and keen to change if things are not working
- Develop teams and a network of support
- Do not feel alone; talk about your stress
- Set aside time for personal development and continuous education
- Attend training and courses that will increase your knowledge and skills
- Seek guidance on careers and examination preparation
- Have a healthy diet
- Find time for activities or hobbies you really enjoy
- Celebrate success and accomplishment
- Book annual leave in advance and organize a holiday – look forward to it

Worked examples

'Coping with pressure' questions can be difficult to answer and are likely to come up during ST recruitment, both on the written application form and during interview. Often questions on coping with pressure may not be directly phrased as such. For example, you may be asked to describe a time when you had to deal with a difficult situation or deal with conflict. Each deanery may word the question slightly differently. It is vital that you understand the question before you begin your answer. Think about what skills the assessor is looking for and what you need to demonstrate.

Examples do not need to be glamorous, but they need to demonstrate a reflective, organized and thoughtful approach. This tells those shortlisting that you would cope with the greater pressures of further training.

 Give an example of a situation when you felt under pressure. How did you manage this and what did you learn that will be relevant to your specialty training?

There are three distinct parts to this question and you must address each part. Ensure that you keep referring back to the question as you write your answer to make sure that you answer it all.

Start off by thinking about potential examples that may be suitable. The example could be from a clinical or non-clinical setting. To help you choose the most suitable example, select the one with a clear and definable outcome, which allows you to demonstrate your skills and reflect on what you have learnt. Remember you will be marked on how you coped under pressure rather than the situation itself, so overly dramatic examples will not help you to gain marks. Avoid examples that could show yourself or colleagues in a negative light and avoid criticizing the system or colleagues. Aim to select an example that ends with a satisfactory outcome. Ideally the example should be from the specialty you are applying for – that is a medical example if applying to Core Medical Training. Suitable examples may include dealing with a difficult patient or relative, juggling several deadlines, personal difficulties or setbacks, handling criticism or feeling out of your depth during a particular task. Whichever example you use, make sure you show insight into what the problem was and use it to demonstrate your suitability for ST.

Reflect and evaluate what you have learnt because it will add a personal element to your answer and demonstrates that you can think laterally about a particular situation.

Controversial response

I found myself under enormous pressure with financial strain when the banding for my job was unexpectedly reduced. I had to meet mortgage repayments, in addition to preparing for the forthcoming birth of our child. To help supplement my income, I commenced employment as a taxi driver while balancing my professional and personal life. I learnt to develop my prioritisation and time management skills. I also registered with a locum agency and regularly undertook locum work. As a locum I have learnt to quickly adapt to different environments and it instilled within me the importance of responsibility and accountability which are necessary skills I have for specialty training.

At the time, I was very upset and angry with the Trust and organized meetings to discuss the banding situation with senior management. I have learnt to communicate tactfully and be diplomatic. I will carry these skills forward into my specialty training when communicating with patients and colleagues.

Be very cautious with any controversial or dangerous examples of pressure. There is negativity in this example and it is emotive. Aim to avoid examples where a negative outcome occurred or a patient came to harm. Nevertheless the answer addresses each part of the question. The candidate identifies the stressor and the solution and reflects on what was learnt.

Good response

During my Cardiology post at St Elsewhere's, I was responsible for 30 ward patients, CCU and outlying patients. The number of patients was too high and I found myself under enormous pressure to juggle everything. I liaised with the Specialty Registrar to organize 'split' ward rounds around their clinic timetables and attended nursing handover to identify unwell patients and issues needing immediate attention. I organized my time efficiently, allocating times to each ward used the computer network to reduce geography based problems. I formed a team with another doctor, delegating administrative tasks as appropriate and prioritizing critical issues. Furthermore, I attended weekly teaching with the multidisciplinary team meetings. This has helped me cope with the pressure of the post and spend more time talking and discussing issues with patients. The nursing staff approved of my ability to cope and I was happy in my post.

This is not a glamorous example, but it demonstrates that the applicant can manage pressure by using the multidisciplinary team, managing their time and modifying their behaviour to fit with the environment. The applicant gives the impression of being a hard worker and will get on with the job. However, this response only answers parts of the question. The candidate uses a sweeping statement 'pressure to juggle everything' but does not unravel or identify what the exact pressures were. If someone cannot identify the stressors then they cannot begin to be deal with them. It is important for you to clearly and concisely identify the pressure(s).

This answer does not reflect on what was learnt and its relevance to ST. Therefore, approximately **one-third** of the marks are automatically *dropped*.

Key skills to demonstrate when coping with pressure and managing stress:

- Prioritization
- Planning
- Organization
- Communication
- Teamwork
- Problem solving
- Delegation
- Responsibility
- Time management
- Negotiation
- Awareness of limitations
- Insight and ability to ask for help
- Judgement
- Accountability

Describe one example of how you resolved a difficult problem. What skills did you use and what solution was reached? Explain its relevance to your ST.

This question does not immediately present itself as a 'coping under pressure' question. When answering an ST application question, you must ask yourself exactly what the question is asking, what skills it expects you to demonstrate and how these will be relevant to your forthcoming ST.

The example you use can be selected from any setting, but you must describe it concisely. Make sure you clearly display your skills. It is important to include the outcome or solution. However, the way in which you reached that endpoint is more important.

Poor response

While on a busy on-call shift during my last job, I was asked by a colleague to complete feedback forms on his performance. I had not had much experience of working alongside this doctor. However, I had heard from other colleagues that his medical practice was questionable.

I said to him that I had not really worked enough with him and he should seek another colleague. He persisted that he did not have time to find another colleague as his forms were due in the next day and pleaded for me to complete the forms. I felt under pressure and did not feel comfortable. My bleep then sounded. I explained to him that he should have been more organized and not left this until the last minute. I reiterated that I was not in a position to complete the forms. I attended to my bleep and did not complete his forms.

I will carry forward my ability to not give in under pressure and to use my communication skills to provide colleagues with guidance and advice.

This applicant has used an example of pressure from conflict/confrontation. The example also touches on an element of ethical correctness. The answer is not satisfactory because it does not convey the exact manner in which the situation was handled. The applicant appears to have use avoidance tactics to 'solve' the problem. More adjectives are required to describe exactly how the situation was dealt with. The relevance of the example to ST and skills learnt requires far more detail.

Good response

As a BMA representative for the hospital, I faced pressure from my junior doctor colleagues regarding the abrupt introduction of a new unpopular rota. Colleagues demanded that I seek immediate reversal to the older rota.

I organized a meeting with the junior doctors and formed a written report that I presented to senior consultants and the management. I liaised with the rota coordinator and designed a new European Working Time Directive compliant system that gained universal approval.

This experience enhanced my ability to deal maturely with pressures using patience and diplomacy – essential skills required during Specialty Training. I developed skills to prioritize tasks and produce reports. I enhanced my communication skills at all levels which will be important during my specialty training.

This example answers all three components of the question. In particular, the structure of the answer into three distinct paragraphs helps to highlight this to the marker. The first paragraph succinctly sets the scene and identifies the pressure. The second paragraph describes how the candidate successfully managed the pressure and states the outcome. The candidate demonstrates skills such as prioritization, communication skills, time management and professionalism. Further depth is added to the answer in the final paragraph because it demonstrates the candidate's insight into the skills learnt and the relevance to their ST. This answer is well balanced overall. It correctly dedicates fewer words to describing the situation because the candidate recognizes that the marker is relatively less interested in the exact nature of the situation. More focus is given to how the situation was managed and what was learnt from the experience.

Other related questions in recent application forms include:

• What coping strategies do you use when under pressure?

• What skills do you use and why when faced with a problem or challenge? List the three skills you consider most important and why.

• Describe a situation when you demonstrated your ability to cope under pressure. What did you do well and what could you have done differently?

• Describe a situation when you failed to cope with pressure. What did you learn and how did this improve your ability to cope in the future?

SECTION C
Specialty training interviews

15 Preparing a portfolio

Philip J Smith

Introduction

Portfolio is defined as 'an organized presentation of an individual's education, work samples and skills'. In practical terms, it is a visual presentation of your curriculum vitae (CV) – which you will be required to take with you to your specialty training (ST) interviews. Interviewers will use this opportunity to briefly look through your achievements and to verify information from the application form.

 A portfolio is not an easy commodity to prepare, especially at the last moment. You should have it ready in advance so that time leading up to the interview can be spent more productively.

The portfolio may not be specifically scored at interview, but it can be used to initiate questions, especially around audit, research and personal activities. You should portray your greatest achievements to their advantage to invite questions on topics that display you and your strengths well. Educational portfolios, such as e-portfolios, are vital in assessments (such as ARCPs) and should also be taken to interviews.

- Prepare well in advance
- Keep all your certificates and patients' letters and cards in a safe place
- Ensure that you have evidence in your portfolio of whatever you have stated in your application
- Look around for a suitable portfolio file to hold your information – not too large or too small – your work should fit comfortably
- Prepare a formal CV, place this at the front and follow its structure throughout to display the evidence

Do NOT

- **Leave it all to the last moment**
- **Pile together all your work without structuring it**
- **Try to fit too much in, or leave huge unfilled sections**
- **Make it too long – interviewers will lose interest**

Structure your portfolio in the same order as your CV:

- **Personal details**
- **Degrees** – original certificates and also General Medical Council (GMC) registration
- **Prizes/awards/grants/honours/distinctions**
- **Postgraduate/undergraduate qualifications** (e.g. ALS, ATLS)
- **Publications** – provide a list then print each in full
- **Presentations** – local, national, international – print slides, small versions of poster, even a photograph of you and your poster or conference programme/certificate of attendance
- **Audits** – provide a list then print presentation slides
- **Teaching** – print slides where applicable, a one-page description can be produced if not. Include feedback evidence
- **Courses/conferences attended** – list and display certificates or offer a short description

- **Elective details** – if you are proud of this demonstrate your elective proposal and findings
- **Extracurricular activities/responsibilities** – provide descriptions and evidence such as invitations to events organized or photos.

Additionally include:

- **Copies of your workplace assessments, multi-source feedback, evidence of Foundation training completion or letters confirming training jobs**
- **Log-book of practical skills** – procedures relevant to your specialty
- **Evidence of reflective practice** – informal reflective journal of different events, how you felt, how you coped, what you have learnt
- **Additional health professional and patient feedback** – patients' letters or cards are of special value
- **Professional Development Plan**
  - Your educational goals
  - The time period over which you wish to achieve this
  - How you will know you have achieved this goal.

If you are in the process of completing your membership examinations, you cannot put the letters after your name until you have passed all the examinations and are admitted to the relevant College!

- Behind each certificate in your portfolio, keep a number of photocopies of these, as they will be required for interviews

- Ring or write to your old medical school faculty office for additional copies of degree certificates if yours are framed, etc. – usually a small charge will apply

- Think laterally for evidence of your achievements, photos, invitations, letters of thanks from charities

- Give yourself enough time to prepare well in advance – for most people this will take 1–2 months to ensure all the suggested elements are included

16 Getting ready for the interview

Manoj Ramachandran and Marc A Gladman

Introduction

Your application form may get you shortlisted but to get the job that you want you must interview well. It may seem impossible to be able to demonstrate your suitability for a job within what may be only a 30-minute interview covering a range of different topics. However, everyone will be in the same situation. Those who are best prepared for the interview will have a clear advantage and the best chance of securing the job they want. Furthermore, most deaneries rank successful interviewees according to their interview score so that even if you do get offered a job within a deanery, the highest scoring candidates will get the best jobs.

- READ THE PERSONAL SPECIFICATION – most of the questions will be built around this
- Know your way to the location – there is nothing more stressful than getting lost on the way to an interview and being late
- Get there early (leave plenty of time in case you are delayed)
- Be professional throughout the journey – you may be seated next to your interviewer on your way in!
- Carry the telephone number of the contact person at the interview location with you in case you are running late so that you can ring ahead

- Remember to take all required documents to the interview, such as originals and photocopies of your passport, General Medical Council (GMC) certificate and your publications and portfolio
- Wear appropriate clothes – suits for men and dress or trouser suit for women
- Believe in yourself – be confident and smile

The interview format

Your first task is to find out what the interview involves. You can do this by talking to the named medical personnel/staffing officer in the job advert and quizzing previous successful and unsuccessful candidates. The objective is not to find out which questions are going to come up (you will be very fortunate to find that information out!), but to understand the format and set-up of the interview.

You need to collect the following information:

1. When and where will the interview be held?
2. How long are the interviews and how many interviewers will there be? You need to be aware of how much time you have to sell yourself. Most take the form of a 30-minute session, either three 10-minute stations, two 15-minute stations or one 30-minute interview. Academic interviews may consist of even more panellists who you may have had a chance to meet before the interview to discuss areas of interest. The set-up does vary from deanery to deanery.
3. What is the style of interview? Most interviews are simple face-to face question and answer sessions. Occasionally, you may be expected to prepare a small presentation for the panel on a topic that is either sent to you in advance or given to you on the day. You may also encounter OSCE-style interviews (OSCE stands for Objective Structured Clinical Examination) where you are expected to complete a task, e.g. obtaining consent from a patient model, and you are marked according to strict criteria that the interviewers have to hand. There is an increasing trend towards OSCE-style interviews at all levels in the medical profession, as they are seen as fair, objective

and easily reproducible. Expect the different interview styles such as open-ended questions to explore knowledge, commitments and capabilities; unpredictable and probing questions aimed at provoking a reaction and seeing how the candidate copes under pressure; questions about hot topics in medicine provoking the candidate to express an opinion; and questions based on speciality-specific scenarios.

The interview panel

It may be difficult to work out exactly who is going to sit on the panel (some interviewers may even be recruited in at short notice!) but expect a wide and fair representation of your chosen specialty. In addition to senior medical staff, i.e. consultants, expect an assortment of fellow interviewers. The panel may include lay members of the public, representatives of your Royal College, members of specialty training (ST) committees related to the post and professionals allied to medicine, e.g. practice nurses, physiotherapists and nurse practitioners. They will each have a specific question to ask you and, strictly speaking, they should put the same question to all interviewees in order to objectively compare the answers.

Practise, practise, practise

You must make yourself aware of the common questions that are asked frequently in interviews and then prepare and practise answers to them. It is best to practise in front of a mirror and watch all the verbal and non-verbal cues that you emit. Close to the interview, practise with your formal suit or dress on so that you get used to exactly what it will feel like on the day. You may also find it useful to practise with colleagues and seniors who have been through the interview process on several occasions. Ask their advice on how to answer specific questions and implore them to give you honest feedback on your answers and technique.

If you feel you need further help, you should attend courses specifically aimed at the interview process. Try to choose one that caters for the level or specialty that you are interested in. More importantly, choose a course that offers one-to-one practice and feedback – you will find this invaluable.

Before the interview

There are several points to consider before you step into the interview room.

What should you take?

The following is a list of items that you should consider taking with you to your interview:

- The letter confirming your interview – make absolutely sure you know exactly where the interviews are being held, and a map of the location if you haven't been there before.

- A copy of your curriculum vitae (CV) – often, you are requested to bring this along, but you may also find it helpful to refresh your memory of your previous achievements and to remind yourself of exactly what you have down on your CV. Make a list of the 'big guns' you want to sell and bring this list along too.

- Documents requested by the interview panel – this might include copies of your GMC and educational certificates, course attendance confirmation certificates and copies of your publications. It is worth investing in a leather-bound portfolio with loose leaves into which you can insert the requested documents – this ensures that the documents are easy to handle and retrieve after use, and adds a professional touch.

- Passport photographs – these are often requested by medical personnel/staffing officers.

Getting there

If possible, you should aim to get to the interview location at least 30–45 minutes in advance. Any earlier and you may have to suffer the stress of a prolonged and nervous wait with your fellow interviewees. Any later and you may be cutting it too fine.

Remember that the interviews can often run early or late, and you may be called for at a time that you do not expect – so arrive in good time.

If you have never been to the venue before it may be possible to do a dry run on a day before the interview. Make sure that you listen out for travel updates before you set off on the day itself. If all this sounds obvious, let us assure you that we have met several candidates who have either missed an interview altogether (usually because they had to travel a great distance) or have turned up late. Being late may be excused if you have a good enough reason, but it certainly does not set a good precedent for the kind of trainee that you are going to be.

How to behave

Note that the interview starts the moment you appear within the environs of the venue. As far as you are concerned, you are being watched at all times. There may be people who are part of the interview process (e.g. medical personnel and members of the interview panel) travelling to the venue at the same time as you. If you behave in a manner that is unbecoming (e.g. being rude to fellow passengers on the train – unlikely but not impossible!), this may well be noted.

When you enter the venue itself, there are receptionists and medical personnel/staffing officers who are also watching your every move. Note that the latter pop in and out of the interviews and have direct contact with the interview panel – so watch how you behave in front of them.

You must behave appropriately around the other candidates too. For a nervous candidate, there is nothing more infuriating than a bunch of 'mates' openly discussing the interview, assessing their chances and loudly discussing their lives in the waiting area. Equally, there are those who insist on assessing their competitors' chances by direct questioning. Again, this can be very annoying. Our general advice is that it is safer to be quiet and discreet, particularly when you are being watched at all times. Only speak when you are spoken to and speak as little as possible, concentrating on getting yourself in the right frame of mind for the interview.

Special considerations

You know your body, and you know how it behaves in stressful situations. So be aware of:

- **Perspiration – some people sweat in stressful situations, while others don't. If you are prone to sweating, learn how to control it as much as you can. Make sure that at least your hands are free of sweat when you go in to shake the interviewers' hands. Go to the bathroom and wash and dry your hands immediately before the interview. Another simple technique is to hold the palms of your hand up against your cheeks – the heat emitted from your face can help to keep your hands dry.**

- **Ablutions – suffice it to say that you shouldn't need to ask for the restroom in the middle of the interview.**

- **Posture and presence – make sure you stand up straight when you walk into the interview room. Poise is a difficult characteristic to teach but it is something you must be aware of.**

- **Smile – smile often and appropriately! Do not smile inanely at the interviewers just because you feel the need to smile constantly.**

- **Don't forget to switch off pagers, bleeps, mobile phones and any other electronic or communication devices before you walk in.**

General appearance

Think hard about what you will be wearing to the interview. Stand in front of a mirror and look at yourself from top to bottom.

1. Hair – for men, make sure your hair is kept neat, trimmed and under control. For women, it's a matter of personal preference but as a general rule, control of your hair is more important than the exact style, appearance or length. Try not to fiddle with your hair during the interview – this may be interpreted as a sign of nervousness.
2. Personal hygiene – make sure you have thought about the length of your fingernails, dandruff, body odour and breath. Try not to flood the interview room with your favourite perfume or aftershave.
3. Handshake – use a firm handshake (not too soft or hard) and importantly, only shake hands with an interviewer *if they offer their hand to you*. It can be interpreted as quite aggressive to enter the room and offer your hand immediately to all the interviewers.

The following are general rules only: ultimately, it is your decision what to wear – go with what makes you feel confident on the day and preferably choose something that you have worn before and are comfortable in.

Score maximization at interview

We again urge you to re-read Chapter 5 of this book as you begin your interview preparation. All the same considerations apply when preparing for the interview. You must be extremely focused and have your big guns, and examples that demonstrate them, ready in mind so that you can communicate these to the panel. Once the panel have asked you to 'tell us about a recent example that demonstrates your ability to work in a team' this is *not* the time to start searching the depths of your memory for a suitable example. Instead, you should be poised like a sprinter on the starting blocks waiting to leap into action with your structured, organized answer.

Q: What is the purpose of the interview and what are my main aims during it?

A: The interview provides the panel with the opportunity to again seek evidence of specific academic achievements and clinical and non-clinical skills. Importantly, therefore, it is **your** opportunity to:

- *sell yourself – deliver an 'Oscar-winning performance'*

- *demonstrate possession of the skills that the panel are seeking – 'give them what they want'*

- *stand out from the crowd*

- *secure your dream job!*

Be sure to keep these objectives in mind while preparing for the interview, and more importantly, during the interview itself as you are delivering your responses

Prepare for the interview in **exactly** the same way as you did for the application form. Consider the interview as an 'oral' version of the application form. Consequently, you will need to demonstrate to the interview panel that you possess the necessary skills to gain entry to ST. However, this time you must do it verbally with spoken instead of written word.

It may sound obvious, but unless you adequately demonstrate (and communicate to the panel!) **satisfactory attainment** of the skills sought during the interview, you will not pick up the points on offer and thus you will **not** get appointed.

All too often applicants are relieved to have merely survived the interview. This should **not** be your aim. Instead, your aim should be to **excel and stand out from the crowd.**

Preparing your responses

It is no exaggeration to say that appropriate preparation for an interview takes many hours. We usually try to book a couple of days of annual leave before an interview to sit down and prepare our responses. With the aid of this book, and by talking to colleagues who have gone through the process, you should be able to predict just about every question that you can be asked at interview. Therefore, there is absolutely *no* excuse for not having an organized, excellent response ready when asked. Read Chapter 5 again to gain some pointers about a general approach to maximize the scores that you obtain for each question. Crucially, you must structure every response that you give to the panel, just as you would structure your responses during an oral examination. Again, we recommend using the SPAR technique to structure your answer whenever appropriate.

Lack of preparation of responses leads to:

- Blurting out unprepared, ill-considered and disorganized answers, which reflects extremely badly on you

- Excessive 'umming' and 'ahhing' when delivering your responses

- Long periods of very uncomfortable silence while you try desperately to come up with a suitable example to answer the question

---

How your performance will be scored at interview

It is important to have insight into how you are going to be scored by your interviewers. The best way of predicting how interviews will be scored in the future is to look at how they were scored in the past. On the basis of previous scoring sheets, candidates are marked on negative and positive indicators on a scale from 0 to 4, marking how people respond to questions.

Q: How is performance assessed at interview?

A: The interview panel are looking for demonstrable evidence of the skills/characteristics under scrutiny. The scores are based on the relative proportion of positive and negative indicators that you mention during the interview. Typically:

- 0 = No evidence – No evidence reported by candidate

- 1 = Poor – Little evidence of specified positive behavioural indicators; mostly negative indicators displayed, many of which decisively

- 2 = Areas of concern – Limited number of specified positive behavioural indicators displayed; many negative indicators displayed, one or more decisively

- 3 = Satisfactory – Satisfactory display of specified positive behavioural indicators; some negative indicators displayed, but not clearly and decisively

- 4 = Good to excellent – Strong display of specified positive behavioural indicators (and possibly others); few negative indicators displayed, and these considered minor in status

Summary

- Prepare well in advance of your interview.

- Tasks you should consider include finding out in advance about the format of the interview and the interview panel, and preparing an overall strategy in your approach to the specialty interview process.

- Make sure you think carefully about what items to take with you to the interview, what to wear on the day and how to behave when you get there.

- Ensure that you have considered the likely questions and have prepared suitable responses in advance, using your 'big guns' that demonstrate the skills being assessed.

- Think about how to score well in your interview by considering positive and negative aspects of your answers.

17 Generic interview questions

Philip J Smith, Elizabeth A Owen,
Mark J Portou, Manoj Ramachandran
and Marc A Gladman

Introduction

Most specialty interviews cover at least three of the following generic themes:

1. Clinical/non-clinical skills
2. NHS management/political topics
3. Academic skills

The available marks are distributed fairly evenly across these three themes. In this chapter, we will endeavour to demonstrate examples of questions that are commonly asked at interview, and to provide sample answers. For specialty-specific questions, we refer you to Section D of this book, where you can find additional common questions related to the specialty to which you are applying.

 If you do not have numerous publications/presentations, you can claw back marks by wooing the panel with an in-depth knowledge and understanding of current political topics in the NHS and by talking about the skills that you have acquired from your participation in audit and research projects.

1. Clinical/non-clinical skills

Traditionally, clinical knowledge was only ever assessed in postgraduate examination. However, questions related to your clinical skills, judgement and acumen have now crept into interviews. In addition, the interview provides another opportunity to assess (this time face-to-face rather than on an application form) whether you possess the numerous non-clinical skills that are ubiquitous in the personal specifications across all specialties. You can expect that one-third of the interview will be devoted to determining whether you make the grade with respect to your clinical and non-clinical skills.

Q: What specific skills are the panel trying to assess in the clinical/non-clinical skills section of the interview?

A: In this section of the interview, the panel will be assessing your:

- commitment to your speciality

- clinical skills, e.g. problem solving, situational testing

- empathy and communication skills

- ability to cope under pressure

- prioritization skills

- organization and planning skills

As we have stated continuously throughout this book, you must prepare for this section of the interview and be able to deliver slick, powerful answers that will leave a lasting impression on the panel, ensuring that you pick up maximum marks and secure the job that you are after!

- **You would not dream (we hope!) of sitting a postgraduate exam without revising, so why would you contemplate attending an interview without adequate preparation.**

- **Be prepared to 'study' for the clinical/non-clinical skills section of the interview in *exactly* the same way as you prepare for an exam.**

Some of the non-clinical skills have already been covered in greater detail in Section B of this book and we suggest that you take time to revise this section of the book before the interview. Exactly the same principles apply when delivering your responses at interview as during completion of the application form. In what follows, we will provide examples of the questions that are commonly encountered across all specialties. Specialty-specific questions can be found in the following section of this book (Section D).

Commitment to specialty

This is the perfect time to demonstrate your commitment and aptitude to your specialty; showing off your 'big guns' – the extra sessions you have attended that have provided you with greater insight into your chosen specialty.

The key to demonstrating commitment to your specialty is to tell your STORY:

- **S**ell yourself – no one else will!
- **T**otal commitment – you may have given up annual leave or holidays to pursue additional activities. Previous jobs and experiences may have given you confidence in managing conditions in a particular specialty.
- **O**pportunities seized to gain further insight into your chosen specialty – you may have attended scientific meetings/conferences, spoken to senior colleagues, organized electives, completed higher degrees and if you are lucky published or presented (all the BIG GUNS).
- **R**eflection – the best candidates will give an indication of areas within that speciality where they need/want to improve or gain further interest. Try to demonstrate insight into your chosen specialty. For example, there is no point in choosing a career in acute medicine and expecting a lot of free time!
- **Y**our goals – if you want to become a consultant neurosurgeon with a special interest in medulloblastomas, you can say this, but make it clear how you are going to achieve this and your reasons why. Here you can also state that you are aware of the training opportunities in the deanery/teaching hospitals/district general hospitals (DGHs) (so long as you have researched this) and demonstrate how this will help you develop in this specialty.

Why have you applied for a post in core medical training?

Good response

I have successfully completed my FY rotations and I am a clinically competent FY doctor with a range of clinical and communication skills, as evidenced in my portfolio. I can confidently assess and treat acutely unwell patients and have completed an ALS course utilizing these skills. In my FY posts, I worked in the acute admissions unit, with the care of the elderly team and in A&E. During that time, I throughly enjoyed managing the acutely unwell medical patients, seeing a huge variety of medical presentations, from the HIV-positive patient with liver failure, through to the elderly patient with newly diagnosed lung cancer. This exposure to a variety of illness presentations has developed my interest in this specialty. I enjoy this busy and often pressurized specialty and believe my enthusiastic and energetic nature is best suited to this environment.

I now feel able to commit to medicine, and I am currently revising for my MRCP Part 2 examinations. I have sought opportunities to learn more about acute liver failure, attending additional Hepatology clinics in my spare time, as I felt I needed to strengthen my knowledge in this area. I have developed my organizational and IT skills through research and audits in medically related subjects and presented twice internationally on subjects related to Gastroenterology; the specialty that I hope to ultimately progress into. By securing a CMT job, I would be able to learn more and develop my skills further in medicine and continue pursuing a career in Gastroenterology, engaging in further research and audit.

Problem solving

These questions test your ability to think around problems, detect deeper causative issues, and generate workable solutions that may involve a variety of approaches, ultimately leading to effective decision making. We recommend structuring your answer using the SPAR technique. As you will remember from Chapter 5, you need to demonstrate certain skills to the panel. Include as many positive indicators as possible that demonstrate your problem-solving skills in the 'Action' section.

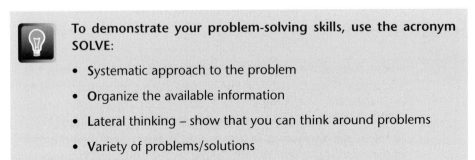

To demonstrate your problem-solving skills, use the acronym SOLVE:

- Systematic approach to the problem

- Organize the available information

- Lateral thinking – show that you can think around problems

- Variety of problems/solutions

- Effective, practical solutions

Describe a situation where you faced a complex problem at work. What did you do to tackle this? What was the outcome? What approach do you use to make decisions?

Poor response

[Situation/problem]

Whilst working in A&E, I was faced with a patient with paranoid schizophrenia, who had given verbal intent of a desire to harm himself and others. He was unwilling to stay for treatment. I had to ensure that public safety was preserved, whilst doing the best for my patient; preferably avoiding physical restraint.

[Action]

Initially, I attempted to 'talk the patient down'. This was unsuccessful, so I alerted the nursing staff and simultaneously enlisted the help of my seniors, the patient's GP and CPN, and the A&E security (organization). The safety of the patient was my immediate concern and thus I stayed with him, trying to reassure him that he was safe.

[Result/reflection]

Having won over his trust, we were able to retain him under an 'emergency section' without the need for physical restraint. No harm came to him or the general public. I now have a new found confidence when assessing psychotic patients.

The choice of example didn't really constitute a complex problem at work, more of any everyday occurrence in the emergency department. The candidate does not demonstrate the skills (SOLVE) that the panel are after. The result is weak and there is limited reflection.

Communication skills

When answering questions that test your communication skills, you should yet again structure your answer using the SPAR technique. As you will remember from Chapter 5, you need to demonstrate certain skills to the panel. Again, include as many positive indicators as possible that demonstrate your communication skills in the 'Action' section.

To demonstrate your communication skills, use the acronym LANGUAGE:

- **L**isten to what the patient says

- **A**djust your language, appropriate to the individual

- **N**ote the concerns of the patient

- **G**lobal (holistic) assessment of patient

- **U**nbiased, non-judgemental approach

- **A**ddress the needs of the patient

- **G**et advice from seniors when appropriate

- **E**nvironment control – adjusted to aid communication, e.g. privacy, etc.

Describe a situation when your communication skills made a fundamental difference to the patient. What were the skills you demonstrated and how did they affect the outcome?

Good response

[Situation/problem]

An intravenous drug abuser presented to A&E breathless, pyrexial, with a swollen right leg and an oozing groin sinus. He was aggressive and antagonistic within the department towards the staff while waiting to be seen. As the FY2 doctor I recognized a developing situation with the risk of the patient self-discharging.

[Action]

I asked to speak to him in a quiet part of the department with the senior charge nurse as support. In a non-judgemental manner, I explored his concern that previous confrontations with staff members had jeopardized his current care. Acknowledging this, I reassured him that his welfare was very important, that his previous disputes would not jeopardize his current care, but explained firmly that he must respect the A&E staff who would not tolerate his behaviour. I assessed him clinically, and then explained empathetically his serious current situation without using jargon and maintaining eye contact. I used his chest x-ray as a visual aid. This gained his trust, understanding and respect. He calmed down and stayed in hospital.

[Result/reflection]

He had staphylococcal septicaemia with infective pulmonary emboli. My communication skills and rapport fundamentally changed his actions and behaviour that night.

With more reflection, this could have been an excellent response.

Organization and planning

This type of question in interviews tests your ability to manage time, follow instructions (if appropriate) and balance urgent and important demands, as well as recognizing your limitations and constraints.

To demonstrate your organizational skills, use the acronym ORGANISE:

- **O**ther plans (contingencies) if appropriate

- **R**isk management

- **G**oal setting

- **A**bility to prioritize

- **N**umerous tasks simultaneously (multi-tasking)

- **I**mprove methodology

- **S**tick to time – meet deadlines

- **E**valuate success/failure

Tell us about a non-clinical situation that required you to be organized.

Good response

[Situation/problem]

Whilst working as doctors' mess president in my FY1 year, I organized a charity summer ball to raise money for the local charities allied to the hospital. The aim was to involve the entire hospital in the charity event so as to raise lots of money and raise morale across the hospital.

[Action]

I worked with a number of my FY colleagues as a team, and delegated the numerous roles to each individual, while I was overall organizer and co-ordinator. We invested the doctors' mess money into the event as initial capital to pay for the venue, DJ, and food. We also wrote to local businesses to ask for support with raffle tickets to maximize the money given to charity, our aim being £2000–3000. After initial setbacks in finding a suitable location to host the ball, we managed to get a considerable reduction in cost to hire a venue. I made selling ball and raffle tickets the main priority, aiming to get a broad attendance from around the specialties.

[Result/reflection]

Organizing such a large event in my spare time was very challenging and demanding. Thankfully, the event raised over £5000 for charity as well as repaying the mess funds, and the evening was sold out. I enjoyed working with my colleagues towards this joint goal. With hindsight, we could have raised even more money if we had increased the cost of the raffle tickets, but I was most proud of our team's ability to stick to schedule and ensure the event was very successful.

2. NHS issues and hot political topics

Questions on NHS issues have repeatedly appeared at the interview stage of the selection process, and tend to account for up to one-third of the entire interview.

Structuring an answer

All your answers should have a logical structure. There are many different ways of approaching questions on the NHS and hot political topics. You may be able to apply the SPAR technique (e.g. when providing examples of how you have been involved with clinical governance), but it is likely that you will need an alternative strategy for this section of the interview.

We recommend the following particularly useful method for tackling questions on the NHS and hot political topics:

- Provide the panel with a brief definition/explanation of the subject

- Explain the 'pros' of the issue as you see them

- Explain the 'cons' of the issue as you see them

- Finally, give a brief personal opinion in light of the 'pros' and 'cons'

What comes up?

The following is by no means meant to be an exhaustive list of what you might be asked, but will give you a flavour of this section of the interview. We will provide some background information for each topic, so that you may incorporate this into the definition/explanation that you give to the panel. It should also provide some insight into the pros and cons of the topic in question.

The NHS

What do you know about the organization of the NHS?

The NHS is the publicly funded health-care system of the UK. It was conceived on 5 July 1948 with the aim of providing health-care for all, which was free at the point of delivery. The creation of the NHS saw the nationalization of hospitals, and their running through a regional framework of control. The NHS has grown to become the largest organization in Europe, and the third or fourth largest in the world, employing around 1.5 million people. Its structure in England is illustrated in Figure 17.1.

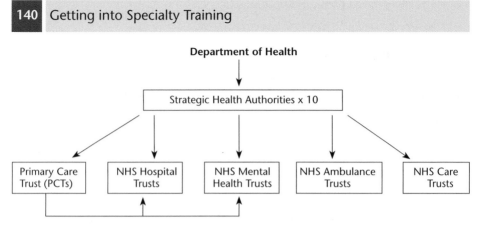

Figure 17.1 Current NHS structure in England.

Strategic Health Authorities (SHAs)

These were created in 2002 to replace the previous NHS health authorities. They are responsible for managing and setting the strategic direction of the NHS locally. They also oversee the local health services, ensuring their quality and performance, and are responsible for increasing the capacity of these local health services. SHAs implement national health agendas, such as cancer services, into the local health services. SHAs essentially link the Department of Health (DoH) with the rest of the NHS.

Primary Care Trusts (PCTs)

These have been in place since 2002 and report directly to their local SHAs. There are currently 152 PCTs in England. Nationally PCTs handle approximately 80% of the total NHS budget, and as local individual organizations they have their own budgets and set their own local priorities. They directly provide a range of community health services, and fund general practice and medical prescriptions. PCTs also commission secondary hospital and mental health services from NHS trusts or occasionally the private sector.

The Healthcare Commission

Which bodies exist to monitor standards in the NHS?

This sample question demonstrates that it may not always be entirely obvious that the panel are asking about a particular organization.

The Healthcare Commission is an independent body formed in April 2004 to replace the Commission for Healthcare Improvement (CHI) and assuming some responsibilities of the National Care Standards Commission and the Audit Commission.

Q: What are the aims of the Healthcare Commission?

A: These include:

- Driving improvement in the standards of health care delivered by the NHS
- Assessment of the performance of each NHS trust in England
- Publication of this assessment in the form of an annual 'health check' (which replaced the previous 'star rating' system)
- Independent review of complaints that are unable to be resolved locally
- Investigation of serious failures in the provision of health care

Pros

- Provides annual health checks on trusts to grade performance
- Ensures standards are met
- Provides mechanism for management of serious complaints
- Investigates serious clinical incidences.

Cons

- Frequent name/role changes since original implementation
- Increased layer of bureaucracy.

Clinical governance

Q1. Tell me about your experience of clinical governance and how does it affect your practice?

Q2. What is your understanding of the role of clinical governance within the NHS?

This topic is covered in greater detail in Chapter 9 of this book.

The seven 'pillars' can be helpfully memorized using the acronym SPARE IT:

- **S**taffing and staff management
- **P**atient and public involvement
- **A**udit
- **R**isk management
- **E**ffectiveness and research
- **I**nformation technology
- **T**raining and education

National Institute for Health and Clinical Excellence (NICE) (http://www.nice.org.uk)

What is the role of NICE? What do they do?

NICE is the independent organization responsible for providing national guidance on the promotion of good health and the prevention of ill health. It was established in 1999 (and in 2005 merged with the Health Development Agency) to standardize the provision and availability of health care in the UK on the basis of efficacy and cost-effectiveness.

NICE produces guidance on three aspects of health care:

- Public health (health promotion)
- Health technologies (new drugs, cost-effectiveness, safety of interventions)
- Clinical practice (clinical guidance based on current best evidence).

Pros

- Centralized body of experts examines best available evidence
- Provides clinical and economic evaluation of new treatments
- Provides guidelines to ensure national minimum standards of care
- Attempts to address health inequalities
- Aims to protect public resources against spiralling cost of health care.

Cons

- Restriction on drugs poorly accepted by patients and media
- Strong political influence
- Potential to restrict clinical freedom
- 'Post code lottery' still exists
- Works in national interest and not in best interests of individual patients
- Criticism over potential bias in methods of determining cost-effectiveness
- Approval process not transparent.

Familiarize yourself with at least one guideline or appraisal relevant to your specialty before your interview.

National Patient Safety Agency (NPSA) (http://www.npsa.nhs.uk)

Tell us how patient safety is ensured in the modern NHS?

The NPSA is a division of the DoH responsible for improving patient safety. It has three divisions:

- Patient Safety Division (England and Wales)
- National Clinical Assessment Service (England, Wales and Northern Ireland)
- National Research Ethics Service (UK)

The Patient Safety Division collects and monitors patient safety incidents and near misses through a national reporting system (NRLS – National Reporting and Learning System). The National Clinical Assessment Service is an advisory service to those working within the NHS who have concerns regarding the performance of a doctor or a dentist. This service does not regulate or discipline, it simply gives confidential advice to the referrer. The National Research Ethics Service, launched in 2007, offers a UK-wide system of ethical review to protect research participants and comprises the Central Office for Research Ethics Committees (COREC) and Research Ethics Committees (RECs in England).

 The NPSA has recently launched its national 'clean your hands' campaign in an attempt to reduce the spread of hospital-acquired infections.

Pros

- Provides rapid responses to critical incidents
- Analysis of incidents and solutions
- Holds national database of incidents on NRLS
- Provides guidance for local implementation of patient safety measures.

Cons

- 'No blame culture' required for open reporting of incidences slow to develop
- Bureaucratic process, removed from ground level clinical practice
- Implementations and changes slow to manifest.

The Care Quality Commission (CQC) (http://www.cqc.org.uk)

How is quality assessed in the NHS?

This organization essentially assesses the quality of the NHS, private and voluntary health-care services available. It also assesses the provision of NHS services and performs NHS trust 'health checks', publishing health service data. The CQC was previously called the Commission for Health Improvement and then the Healthcare Commission.

The NHS plan

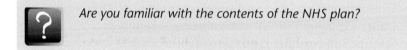

Are you familiar with the contents of the NHS plan?

In July 2000 the DoH published its future vision for NHS reform and service delivery in a document called 'The NHS Plan'.

Q: What are the main points covered in the NHS plan?

A: These include:

- Devolution of power from centralized government (DoH) to local control

- Setting of national standards overseen by new regulatory bodies (CHI – later the Healthcare Commission)

- Role of NICE defined

- Social services amalgamated with the NHS to ensure that both services are commissioned with common purpose

- New consultant and general practitioner (GP) contracts

- Creation of extended practice nursing staff and expansion of nurse consultants
- Patient advocates in every hospital, surveys and forums, and overall increased patient choice
- Private health-care providers utilized at the expense of the NHS to drive down waiting lists
- Maximum waiting times introduced, e.g. maximum 48 hours for a GP appointment and maximum A+E and outpatient waiting times
- Rapid access chest pain clinics
- Improvement in cancer screening programmes and drug availability to be introduced

Pros

- Commitment to large sustained increase in NHS funding
- Large expansion of GP and consultant numbers
- Specific improvements to fundamental patient services such as cancer and ischaemic heart disease.

Cons

- Introduction of controversial targets
- Proposed restrictions on new consultant participation in private sector
- Creation of many new agencies and task forces may further increase NHS bureaucracy
- Unclear how cash injection will be utilized
- Rating systems punish poor performance with less funding
- Use of extended practice health-care professionals controversial
- Local devolution of health government may lead to lack of overall leadership.

The Darzi report

What are the recommendations of the Darzi report?

In June 2008 Lord Darzi, the politically appointed Health Minister, published his final report *'High quality care for all: NHS next stage review final report'*. This report was published to issue a current state of the NHS report around its 60th birthday.

Q: What are the main points covered in the Darzi report?

A: These include:

- Personalization of health-care services

- Focus on health promotion

- Tackling obesity, alcohol harm, drug addiction, reducing smoking, improving sexual health and improving mental health

- 'Reduce your risk' campaign for vascular risk

- Pilot personal loans – patients managing own health-care budgets

- Creation of 150 GP-led 'health centres' nationally

- 100 new GP practices in the most deprived areas

One of the most controversial ideas raised within this report was the concept of 'polyclinic' health centres. The creation of these large health centres, replacing many smaller GP practices, was suggested to increase the scope of the service provided in primary care and to move towards a 'shift of services out of hospital settings'. The polyclinic model for the future of primary care is intended to be trialled in London, and eventually rolled out across the country.

'Polyclinics'

Pros

- Extended opening hours
- Greater accessibility
- Offer secondary care services such as antenatal and postnatal care, and some specialty services.

Cons

- Lack of continuity – end of doctor–patient relationship
- Centralized location – may decrease physical accessibility
- Threatens position of smaller hospitals.

Good medical practice

What constitutes good medical practice?

In November 2006, 'Good Medical Practice', a document outlining the duties of a doctor, was produced by the General Medical Council. While it is essential to be familiar with this document, it is not a list of statutory rules and clinical judgement. It should be used to adapt to various situations that a doctor could encounter. Essentially, a patient must be able to trust a doctor with both their health and their life. To justify that trust and fulfil their role, doctors must show respect for human life and exhibit an acceptable degree of professionalism.

The seven key areas of Good Medical Practice:

- Good clinical care
- Maintaining good medical practice
- Teaching and training, appraising and assessing
- Relationships with patients
- Working with colleagues
- Probity
- Health

3. Academic issues

During this 10-minute section of the interview, you can reasonably be expected to be quizzed on your knowledge and experience of:

- audit and research
- teaching.

Many of the basic principles and key concepts relating to these subjects have already been covered in Chapters 7 and 8 of this book and you are urged to review this information again. Furthermore, the application form questions posed in these chapters could easily (or alternatively) be asked during the interview. Accordingly, discussion of *'what is your experience of audit/research/teaching'* will not be covered again in this chapter to avoid repetition.

Once again, it is critical to demonstrate to the panel that you fully appreciate and have an in-depth understanding of these topics. More importantly, you must be able to communicate the skills that you have acquired from participating in such activities (i.e. 'give the selectors what they want') and reflect upon these new skills and their relevance to your training.

Audit and research

 What is the difference between audit and research?

In simplistic terms, research tells us what we SHOULD be doing. Audit determines whether we ARE doing what we should be doing in everyday clinical practice. Alternatively, research is based on a hypothesis and aims to create new knowledge (*creates a gold standard*), while audit is the process of *comparing* current or local practice to a gold standard.

 How do you go about setting up a research project?

They want to know that you are aware of the main elements and considerations that are involved in good research, here are a few:

- Defining clearly your objectives and hypothesis
- What kind of trial (that you know the levels of evidence – covered later)
- Ethical considerations and approval and confidentiality
- Define the population and recruitment of subjects, including informed consent
- How data would be collected
- Analysis of results and conclusions and possibility of leading to further research
- What will happen to the data and results, knowing that it's unethical to leave research unfinished and unpublished
- If you would stop the trial at any point
- That you would write up for publication.

How does audit benefit the trust?

It is worth mentioning the following:

- Clinical and financial benefits
- Identifies and promotes good practice – improves patient care
- Leads to improvements in service delivery and outcomes
- Promotes efficiency by ensuring a better use of resources; this may mean the trust can gain a better reputation and also rationalize expense
- Many targets are given financial incentives, e.g. 18-week wait for outpatient clinic appointments, and some contribute to the inspection score a trust is awarded
- It can be used as evidence and to provide information to relevant institutions about the effectiveness of their service
- Facilitates budget planning and application, allowing justification of services
- Provides opportunities for training and education, and is a requirement for clinical governance

What levels of evidence do you know about?

Try to keep the answer to this question simple and avoid getting tied up in the specific detail of the complicated systems for defining levels of evidence. The Centre for Evidence-Based Medicine, Oxford (www.cebm.net) contains the strict definitions. Evidence is ranked according to its strength, 1a to 5, with 1a being the 'best quality'. The NHS and clinical guidelines tend to use an A–D categorical classification, based on the same system.

Levels of evidence may be summarized as follows:

Level 1: Strong evidence from systematic reviews, meta-analysis of multiple randomized controlled trials (RCTs) and high quality single RCTs

Level 2: Systematic review of cohort studies, high quality cohort studies, low quality RCTs

Level 3: Systematic review of case-control study and individual case–control studies

Level 4: Case-series and poor quality cohort and case–control studies

Level 5: Expert opinion without explicit critical appraisal, or based on physiology, bench research or first principles

Do you think all trainee doctors should do research?

This is a potentially contentious question and the member of the panel asking it may hold a biased view (compare the opinion of a professor versus a 'jobbing' DGH consultant!). Essentially, there is *no* right or wrong answer and the panel (yet again!) wants to assess your knowledge of the topic and the more lateral issues associated with it.

Q: How do I tackle such a potentially contentious question and appease the varying opinions of the different members of the interview panel?

A: We suggest using the **three Cs** in this situation:

- Consider both sides of the argument

- Communicate these to the panel

- Cautiously express your own personal view

It is important to demonstrate that you understand that the purpose of research is to advance medical knowledge and thus research is important to all doctors as there is potential to improve the quality of patient care. However, the degree of interest is variable between doctors, with some being purely researchers, others purely clinical and the others a combination of the two. Further, you should acknowledge (as detailed in Chapter 8) that participation also enables new skills to be acquired.

Q: What are the pros and cons of research?

A: Pros:

- First-hand experience of principles and practices of research

- Generic skills gained (see Chapter 8)

- Career progression and development of a specialist field of interest

- Possibility of adding new and important information to the clinical field

Cons:

- No value in poor research of unrelated interest, if individual is not motivated or supported

- Time spent away from clinical practice

- Generic skills can be gained in other ways

- Can learn to appraise and apply research of others without having first-hand experience

You can include reference to your personal experience and use this opportunity to emphasize your achievements. If you have had a paper published or presented at a conference, say so. If you got a first class degree, tell them. You will not be asked directly and they won't necessarily look at your form. Reflection is crucial – what does your experience add to your personal profile? How has it made you a better doctor? You may be asked why you chose to do a BSc or not. Again the actual answer is not as important as the reflection and what you gained from this experience or your plans for the future.

 Talk about a recent paper you have read and how it changed your practice.

It is useful to talk about a paper that you may have presented at a journal club as you have probably gone into a lot of detail and know it well. Remember, this is a specialty training (ST) interview, so pick a paper that has high relevance to your chosen specialty.

Apply the SPAR technique.

[Situation]

I read a paper presenting the finding of the PIVOT trial, which was a multi-centre randomized controlled trial comparing oral amoxicillin and IV benzylpenicillin in community acquired pneumonia in children.

(Problem: what is important about this research?)

It's an important area to research because pneumonia is very common, the oral route is preferable for children (parents and doctors) and the BTS guidelines of 2002 were based on a consensus recommendation, not evidence, as trials were not available.

[Action: what were the results of this trial?]

Their outcome measure was the time taken for resolution of pyrexia. They also looked at how long the children required oxygen and how long they stayed in hospital. Complications of pneumonia were also noted and if the children needed further treatment and how long a full recovery took. They found that there was equivalence for resolution of temperature but the IV group stayed in hospital and required oxygen longer, there were similar complication rates in each group. Their conclusion was that oral amoxicillin and IV benzylpenicillin have equivalent efficacy for treating pneumonia in previously well children and that oral treatment allowed children to go home sooner and avoided the pain of cannulation.

[Reflection: what were the good and bad aspects of this research and how did it change your practice?]

I thought this was a good trial because it was randomized and had a large number of patients, the inclusion and exclusion criteria were sensible. It was pragmatic which meant the children did not stay in hospital longer or receive extra treatment due to the trial, it added important information on a topic that is very relevant and where evidence is lacking. After my presentation of this paper in a journal club meeting, our department decided that first line treatment in all but the sickest children should be oral amoxicillin, even if oxygen and admission were required.

Teaching

Almost every ST interview will have at least one question dedicated towards teaching and so it is worth thinking about how you may prepare for these questions.

Typical questions encountered during recent rounds of interviews include:

- *What is your experience of teaching?*

- *What is the most effective method of teaching for doctors in training?*

- *What techniques do you use when you're teaching a specific skill?*

- *How can doctors improve their teaching abilities?*

- *Some people say that all doctors should teach, do you agree?*

- *What are the qualities of a good teacher?*

Depending on how this question is phrased, you will need to demonstrate that you are conversant with different styles of teaching and can deliver slick examples that convey this knowledge.

We recommend the use of the acronym VARIOUS

- **V**ariety of formats and audiences – didactic vs interactive; problem-based vs lecture-based; bedside vs large group teaching; clinical and non-clinical

- **A**ttendance of courses, e.g. training the trainers, etc.

- **R**eflection on the feedback that you receive

- **I**nformation technology – you need to demonstrate competence with multimedia educational techniques

- **O**bjective appraisal of your teaching abilities – collect feedback/be open

- **O**pen to other teaching methods/techniques

- **U**nderstand that people learn in different ways

- **S**how flexibility of techniques employed, e.g. 'thought showering' (previously called brain storming!); 'cliff-hangers' (a scenario that leaves the group with the important decision to make). Sort out areas of improvement – demonstrate that you are keen to improve your teaching, i.e. attendance

What experience of delivering teaching do you have?

Sample response

On my current medical firm, I have organized small and large group formal Problem Based Learning (PBL) interactive sessions for students and FY doctors, using PowerPoint and diagrammatic illustrations. Weekly bedside and ward-based sessions have developed their history and examination skills. I involve the groups in my teaching by giving them scenarios in which they have to determine patient management.

I have sought feedback from my students, which I have within my portfolio. Students have particularly enjoyed case-based discussions. They also suggested additional handouts (where appropriate) for my sessions. I reflected on their feedback, acknowledged that people learn in different ways and have made the changes they suggested. I have had improved feedback since making these changes.

Through completing the 'Teaching the Teachers' course, I have attempted to improve my teaching further and also used the skills learnt on this course to teach nursing staff and other health professionals on the wards and in formal teaching sessions.

SECTION D
Specialty-specific questions

18 Core medical training

Luke Moore and Philip J Smith

Commitment to a medical career

 Please outline your career to date and show how your experiences have contributed to your professional development and to your application for a post as a Core Medical Trainee.

Sample response

After graduating in 2008 with MBChB with Merit and a first class intercalated BSc in Physiology, I developed a keen interest in internal medicine. I further consolidated this interest during my Elective in Samoa, where I intimately assisted in running a Cardiology Clinic for two months, developing my diagnostic and communication skills in this field. Following this I secured a two year Foundation Rotation incorporating posts across two Teaching Hospitals. During this time I actively sought experience in a wide variety of specialties to further my clinical ability, involving myself in additional clinics and amongst other activities organizing time in the Coronary Intervention Laboratory. Work Place Based Assessments and appraisals throughout my Foundation Years have acknowledged my competence as a diagnostician as well as my ability in the practical aspects of internal medicine and my communication skills. I have also actively maintained my academic drive throughout these posts. I have undertaken numerous audits and have recently sought and obtained Research and Ethics Committee approval for a pilot study investigating lung function in the elderly. These experiences have made me an excellent candidate for Core Medical Training and in due course I aim to pursue a career in Cardiology.

Give brief details under separate headings of the clinical experience you have obtained in your posts to date. Please summarize the duties involved, on-call experience and any other details of skills acquired. This may include experience of teamworking and examples of leadership skills you have acquired.

Sample response

FY1 Rotation:

During this year I acquired clinical skills and experience in a busy Teaching Hospital across three intensive specialties – Respiratory Medicine, Haematology and Upper Gastro-Intestinal surgery. During these posts I played an active role in professorial and in autonomous ward rounds, in outpatient clinics and in undertaking a multitude of clinical procedures including (amongst others) chest drains and paracentesis as evidenced by my Work Place Based Assessments. I also gained valuable experience whilst on take during my 1 in 8 on call rota, admitting patients to both internal medicine and to a wide variety of surgical specialties.

FY2 Rotation:

I consolidated the skills and attributes I had acquired during the previous year during my FY2 rotation – comprising Renal Medicine, A&E and Primary Care with a robust on call commitment in each specialty. Whilst in Nephrology, I grasped opportunities to consolidate my practical skills including central venous access, and took an active role in leadership – encouraging commitment and work ethos into the FY1 doctors on the firm and in addition taking charge of programmed teaching periods for the undergraduate medical students. Within my Primary Care placement I undertook an active role in multi-disciplinary team meetings, not only developing an understanding of team-working and roles of individuals but also developing an understanding both of chronic disease management and of the importance of dialogue between primary and secondary/tertiary care. During this year I have further developed my clinical skills through successfully completing both an ALS and an ATLS course.

Please tell us why you want a career in this specialty and what sub-specialty interests you have? What attributes do you have that make you suitable? How have you shown your commitment? You may include any other information not covered elsewhere that you feel will support your application, e.g. administrative contributions, or experience outside medicine.

Sample response

I have aimed to pursue a career in internal medicine, and more specifically Thoracic medicine since my undergraduate period. After graduating with both MBChB and a First Class Intercalated degree in Physiology (during which I published on pulmonary metallo-proteins in a peer reviewed journal) I successfully completed a comprehensive Foundation Year programme encompassing a wide variety of medical specialties. This included four months in a tertiary Professorial Thoracic Medicine unit. There, I not only undertook teaching and autonomous ward rounds, became competent at a diverse range of practical procedures and assisted in outpatients clinics, but also conducted an audit presented at a regional conference and published an abstract on the use of peak flow recordings in acute medical units. Over and above my clinical commitments, I was elected to the post of President of the Doctor's Mess, where I was able to obtain valuable management experience through my work on various Trust committees. Over this period workplace based assessments and appraisals have all complimented me on my attention to detail and my superlative communication skills and it is these, combined with my solid clinical and academic grounding that make me more than suited for a career in internal medicine.

Please give details of your experience in undertaking acute unselected take and the follow-up of admitted patients. List the number of months spent in undertaking acute unselected take.

Sample response

During my two year Foundation Rotation I completed 16 months of acute unselected takes on a 1 in 8 rota. Patients I admitted were reviewed on the Consultant post take ward round allowing case based discussion and could be followed up throughout their admission. This encompassed not only acute medical patients but also unselected surgical patients, thus broadening my experiences of acute presentations to take forward to internal medicine as a specialty.

During this period I have become proficient at managing acute takes having had opportunity on occasion to act up as a middle grade, and also in leading cardiac-arrests. I have developed my technical skills to meet the Core Curriculum and I am independent in many practical procedures as outlined. My experiences as a Foundation doctor have developed my ability to participate in outpatient clinics and be confident in all aspects of inpatient care including care of the critically ill, autonomous ward rounds and multi-disciplinary meetings. These competencies are evidenced by workplace based assessments and appraisals throughout the rotation. My knowledge and clinical acumen are supported by my achieving full MRCP (UK).

Clinical skills

Questions testing your knowledge in medicine tend to be reserved for the interview. Often a station is dedicated to this and it may take the form of a mini-viva. You will often be given a stem, and the interviewer may prompt you according to your response and your progress.

Common clinical scenarios in the interview include:

- Confused elderly patient
- Diabetic ketoacidosis presenting as abdominal pain
- Hypoglycaemia – Addisonian crisis
- Left-sided weakness/neurological insult
- Unexplained weight loss investigated
- Shortness of breath secondary to cardiac or respiratory causes.

The following worked scenario is typical of the ones you may encounter in the interview.

You are the specialty training (ST) doctor on call at night, and are called to see a 74-year-old man on the care of the elderly ward who has become confused and aggressive on the ward. He was admitted 2 days ago after a mechanical fall at home. What do you do?

'The first thing I would like to do is check that the patient is stable and check his airway, breathing and circulation are all stable.'

All of his observations are stable, but he is still confused and the nurses report that the night before he was settled and slept all night.

'I would like to find out some more history from the patient and examine him thoroughly, including a mental state examination, and review his investigations to date ensuring that I exclude some important causes of acute confusion such as sepsis, silent myocardial infarction (MI), stroke, pain, hypoxia, hypoglycaemia, retention, alcohol withdrawal, and iatrogenic drug causes.'

So from the notes, you see that the man had a mental state examination score of 10/10 on admission, but now it is 8/10. His blood sugar is normal. In his notes it says he fell over a piece of carpet at home, and was noted to drink up to two bottles of spirits per day. All his inflammatory markers were normal on admission. He has no other significant history or past medical history, he is passing urine, and there are no other focal examination findings, apart from some left hip pain.

'Well assuming he was not on any medication for alcohol withdrawal, I would ensure he received the necessary multivitamin and benzodiazepine treatment, not ignoring the other remaining differentials that have to be excluded. I would thoroughly examine his left hip for any evidence of having a fractured neck of femur. I would also ask the nurses if there has been any history of a fall as an inpatient. I would ask for the patient to be nursed in a well-lit room and send off some routine bloods, ask for an ECG to exclude a silent MI and get an urgent X-ray of his hip, while prescibing analgesia for his pain.'

The ECG is normal, but the X-ray of his left hip shows a left fractured neck of femur, also the pelvic bones have multiple sclerotic lesions throughout.

'Then I would inform the orthopaedic team that the patient has fractured his neck of femur as well as my registrar, and ensure he has TED stockings on as well as other DVT prophylaxis such as low molecular weight heparin. I would then ensure the man's haemoglobin has not dropped from his injury, send off a bone profile to check his calcium level which if high could also make him confused and treat him with i.v. fluids and bisphosphonates if necessary. I would do a PSA as the lesions in the bone suggest a metastatic carcinoma, probably of his prostate gland. I would also ask the nursing staff to keep a very close observation on the man overnight, and I would inform his medical team of the night's findings in the morning. If the PSA was significantly raised in the context of the previous findings, I would expect the orthopaedic team to be informed so they could take a bone biopsy, and ask the urology team to be involved in his management.'

Thank you very much, we will ask you to stop there and move onto your next station.

Another example scenario is as follows:

A normally fit and well 17-year-old female arrives in Accident and Emergency with her boyfriend complaining of abdominal pain. The nurse tells you she has a mild tachycardia of 100 bpm. She complains of feeling thirsty, and her boyfriend mentions she can't stop going to the toilet. What do you do?

'The first thing I would like to do is ensure her A, B, C, D are dealt with and find out what her blood sugar recording is.'

Her airway is patent and clear, but her respiratory rate is increased at 24 breaths a minute, but her chest is clear and saturation on room air is 98%, her BP is 100/60 and she is mildly tachycardic. Her blood sugar is 26 on two recordings. Her GCS is 13/15 and her abdomen is soft and non-tender.

'Based on the above findings, my concern is that the girl is a newly diagnosed diabetic who may be in diabetic ketoacidosis. I would assure she was in or moved to an appropriate area i.e. resus.

I would also take a focused history and examine her to ensure I did not miss any focus of infection in particular.

At the same time, I would ask for help and ask if someone could place some high flow oxygen on her, as well as placing two large cannulae into her, starting her on fluid resuscitation while I send off some bloods such as FBC, U+E, CRP and blood gas, as well as asking for a pregnancy test and for a measurement of urinary ketones. I would ask the nursing staff to set up a sliding scale and run this according to the hospital's guidelines on managing DKA. I would also want to complete a full sepsis screen including CXR and urinalysis, and blood culture if febrile.'

What is the risk of overly aggressive fluid resuscitation?

'Rapid changes in blood osmolarity can lead to fluid shift and cerebral oedema in worst case scenario. After an initial fluid bolus, I would aim to correct her dehydration over 48 hours and carefully monitor fluid balance – a urinary catheter would be necessary.'

The patient's pregnancy test is negative, but her urinary ketones are extremely high, and her blood gas shows a pH 6.9 with a base excess of –15. Her boyfriend reports that she has lost a lot of weight recently, but is normally fit and well. She now tells you she has felt feverish over the last 2 days, and complains of dysuria. As you are talking to her, she becomes drowsy and agitated.

'So my working diagnosis remains the same, that the girl has diabetic ketoacidosis, she is decompensating, and needs intensive support. I would immediately ask for help, as this girl is at risk of not being able to support her own airway and aspiration and may now require urgent intubation. I would assess her A, B and C again and ask for urgent anaesthetic, and intensive care support, as well.'

The ITU registrar arrives quickly and feels that the patient needs intubation, so intubates her and she is transferred to ITU. What further medical interventions would be advisable based on the information you are aware of?

'I would start the girl on empirical antibiotics, such as cefuroxime, to cover a potential urinary infection. I would also advise her starting on a prophylactic dose of low molecular weight heparin as there is an increased risk of thromboembolic events as well as inserting an nasogastric tube (NGT) because of the risk of aspiration in this setting.'

19 Core surgical training

Marc A Gladman

'A surgeon should be of deep intelligence and of a temperate and moderate disposition; (s)he should be humble, brave, but not audacious. (S)He should have well-formed hands and a strong body. (S)He must be able to train all the members of the team to the capable fulfilment of the wishes of his(her) mind. (S)He should be well-grounded in basic science, and should know not only medicine but every part of philosophy. (S)He should know logic well, so as to be able to understand what is written, to talk properly, and to support what (s)he has to say by good reasons.'
Guido Lanfranchi, *Chirurgia Magna*, 1296

Introduction

Since the 13th century, the personal skills, attributes and qualities required of surgeons have been clearly defined. In the 21st century, selectors are looking to appoint individuals who demonstrate such skills to specialty training (ST) posts in surgery. How to approach many of the 'generic skills' questions has already been covered in greater detail in other sections of this book. In this chapter, I will show you ways in which you can effectively and efficiently communicate that you possess the skills and attributes required for a career in surgery, specifically concentrating on:

- commitment to a surgical career
- clinical skills.

Approach to individual questions

For each question posed, you should ask yourself:

- 'What are they testing?'

- 'What are they after?'

- Only then will you be in a position to 'give them what they want'

Having read Chapters 5, 16 and 17 of this book, you should by now fully appreciate the importance of appropriately structuring your answers. Now is a good time to review the contents of these chapters before you begin tackling specific surgical questions.

Q: What should I be aiming to demonstrate to the selectors to secure an ST post in surgery?

A: You need to demonstrate that you have the potential to develop into and become a surgeon. Therefore you need to:

- Begin to think and communicate like a surgeon – be decisive, logical and methodical when delivering your responses

- Be committed – demonstrate passion for a career in surgery, while also showing insight and awareness of the negative aspects

- Possess sound technical knowledge, clinical expertise and hunger for knowledge

- Demonstrate the required personal skills and attributes

Commitment to a surgical career

The selectors will want to see evidence of not only your *commitment* to a surgical career, but also your *suitability* for such a career. The sorts of questions encountered will thus explore both areas.

What has influenced your decision to follow a career in surgery and why do you think you are particularly suited to it?

Q: *What are they testing?*

A: The selectors are testing your:

- Realistic insight into general surgery
- Appreciation of the demands of a surgical lifestyle
- Knowledge of the training programme
- Understanding of the personal skills/attributes required to be a surgeon

Q: *What are they after?*

A: You need to provide the **six Cs**:

- **C**lear rationale for choosing surgery
- **C**omprehension of surgery and of your own abilities/needs
- **C**areer motivation/goals/development needs
- **C**ommitment to self-development, self-directed learning and reflective/analytical approach to practice
- **C**ritical and enquiring approach to knowledge acquisition
- **C**orroborative information that is relevant and supports rationale/career choice

What has influenced your decision to follow a career in surgery and why do you think you are particularly suited to it?

Sample answer

I decided that I wanted to pursue a career in surgery as an undergraduate. I feel that I am suited to such a career as I enjoy being presented with a problem, identifying and comprehensively considering the available options and then providing a timely solution to it. To confirm my decision, I organized my elective in surgery in a developing country where I was given more responsibility and a more direct role in assisting with patient management and operative surgery. I was impressed watching the surgeons make key decisions under considerable pressure, whilst remaining calm and in control. It also provided me with key insight into the rigors of a surgical lifestyle, and particularly the strong resilience required to identify and correct complications that have arisen as a direct consequence of surgical intervention.

During my FY rotations, I specifically chose to work in acute specialties relevant to surgery. I worked in intensive care, which has given me confidence to manage acutely sick surgical patients with multi-organ dysfunction. During my surgical posts, I have been able to appreciate the importance of prompt action resuscitating sick patients and organizing the staff around me to achieve this. By working on the trauma team, I have learnt the importance of clarity of thought under pressure to achieve accurate diagnoses. I have also been able to identify my own limitations by realising that to gain the most from formal surgical training I should attend a basic surgical skills course to improve my practical skills. I also noted some gaps in my knowledge and addressed this by beginning to study for the MRCS examination. I have joined the Association of Surgeons in Training and have subscribed to the British Journal of Surgery, so that I may keep abreast of important advances in surgical training and knowledge.

Surgeons should be good leaders. Describe, using suitable examples, the skills that you possess that demonstrate that you have potential to be a leader in the future.

Q: What are they testing?

A: In this question, the selectors have taken one of the key attributes of a surgeon (i.e. leadership) and are seeking to establish whether you have the ability to acquire such skills and thus potentially make it as a surgeon.

Q: What are they after?

A: You need to provide the **eight Is** of leadership:

- Intelligence and intellectual flexibility
- Initiative
- Influence
- Integrity
- Information communicator
- Inspiration
- Informality when required
- Improving performance continuously

Surgeons should be good leaders. Describe, using suitable examples, the skills that you possess that demonstrate that you have potential to be a leader in the future. HINT: use the SPAR technique, incorporating the Is of leadership in the 'action' section of your answer.

Clinical skills

'At a given instant everything the surgeon knows suddenly becomes important to the solution of the problem. You can't do it an hour later, or tomorrow. Nor can you go to the library and look it up.'

John W. Kirklin, 1963

Various aspects of your clinical skills may be evaluated:

- Clinical knowledge and expertise
- Technical competence/practical skills
- Situation awareness/judgement under pressure.

BEFORE you go to the interview, it is worth thinking about *all* the common surgical emergencies and how you would answer questions related to them.

The clinical scenarios that you will be presented with will be testing your clinical knowledge, diagnostic skills, ongoing ability to acquire new skills and your technical competence/practical skills.

Clinical knowledge and expertise

It is not possible to go through sample answers for every possible question that could arise, across all of the subspecialties of surgery. However, there are some important points to consider when approaching such questions.

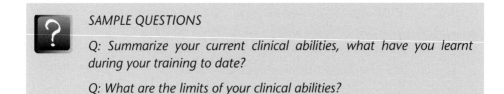

SAMPLE QUESTIONS

Q: Summarize your current clinical abilities, what have you learnt during your training to date?

Q: What are the limits of your clinical abilities?

Q: How can I summarize my clinical abilities/limitations?

A: You should provide a logical, systematic answer. You could divide your abilities into categories as follows:

- emergency/elective
- operative/non-operative
- competent/incompetent
- pre-/intra-/postoperative

SAMPLE QUESTIONS

Q: What are the possible causes and how would you manage a collapsed patient with abdominal pain?

Q: A patient is day 1 following an RTA with multiple long bone fractures. The urine output has been 10 mL for the last 3 hours. What are the possible reasons and what are you going to do?

Q: A 6-year-old boy has a displaced fracture of his radius that requires manipulation. Your registrar is busy in theatre. The accident and emergency registrar has asked you whether you would come and perform the manipulation.

*Q: How should I answer **direct** clinical questions?*

A: You should:

- Predict in advance – they will be on emergencies/key areas of your practice
- Be realistic about what you can manage for your level of training!
- Structure your response as in clinical exams:
  > Resuscitation
  > Assessment
    □ Tests
    □ Treatment (procedures)

When answering clinical questions, do NOT forget to:

- **Ensure patient's safety (and progress from life-saving resuscitation, to assessment, to tests and then treatment)**

- **Keep the patient as the central focus**

- **Keep your response in keeping with your level of experience**

Technical competence/practical skills

SAMPLE QUESTIONS

Q: How many chest drain insertions/appendicectomies/dynamic hip screws/hernia repairs, etc., have you performed?

Q: What level of supervision do you require to perform chest drain insertion/appendicectomy/dynamic hip screw/hernia repair, etc.?

Q: Describe the steps involved in chest drain insertion/appendicectomy/ dynamic hip screw/hernia repair.

Q: How can I summarize my technical abilities/limitations?

A: Again, you should provide a logical, systematic answer. Try to cover:

- Aptitude for practical skills, e.g. hand–eye coordination, dexterity, visuospatial awareness

- Define approximate numbers of procedures/operations

- Describe your level of competency with each procedure/operation (see Top tip below)

- Provide evidence of numbers performed/competency – e.g. validated logbook of procedures, DOPs, etc.

- Attendance at relevant courses, e.g. Basic Surgical Skills

You should define your levels of competency with specific procedures/operations as follows:

- Observed

- Involved with

- Assisted

- Performed under direct supervision, i.e. supervisor present

- Performed under indirect supervision, i.e. supervisor available but not present

- Independent

Summarize the logbook of your procedures/operations.

Situation awareness/judgement under pressure

These questions are designed to assess not only your clinical competence, but also your ability to act under pressure. On application forms you are usually asked to demonstrate such skills by answering an 'open question' (see sample question below). In the interview setting, the questioning can be more dynamic and interactive, tailored to the responses that you provide.

In the interview setting, the panel have much greater flexibility. Be prepared to have to tackle a seemingly unrealistic clinical scenario that is impossible to manage. Frequently, chaos has broken out and there are too many sick patients, with not enough hands on deck! Expect the panel to alter the situation to inject further chaos into the proceedings just as you are getting on top of the 'current' problem and beginning to feel comfortable and in control!

The clinical scenarios that are presented to you (especially by the interview panel) will be assessing your ability to:

- think on your feet

- prioritize

- be flexible with your decision making

- recognize that everyday clinical practice is not static and that patients can deteriorate rapidly in front of you

- anticipate an ever-changing scenario

Most of all they are designed to test:

- whether you can remain calm with ordered rational thought process, enabling you to make accurate, safe clinical decisions in the face of extreme pressure

SAMPLE QUESTIONS

Q: Describe a situation/example from your experience when applying your clinical judgement had a significant impact on patient management. What did you do and how did your judgement contribute to patient health?

Q: Describe a situation where you had to respond quickly to unexpected and stressful circumstances at work. How did you respond?

Q: What are they testing?

A: Your:

- Anticipation of ever-changing clinical scenarios

- Clinical vigilance

- Anticipation of problems

- Awareness of team members

Q: What are they after?

A: Use the acronym **AWARE** to give them what they want:

- **A**lert to signs suggesting deterioration

- **W**ary of potential problems

- **A**ction is taken immediately

- **R**esuscitation principles applied (ALS/ATLS)

- **E**nlist senior/junior help

Describe a situation where you had to respond quickly to unexpected and stressful circumstances at work. How did you respond?

Q: What should I use as suitable examples to demonstrate my judgement under pressure/situation awareness?

A: Suitable examples include:

- Quick decisions required with good reason for no senior help being available

- Pre-emptive escalation in light of your assessment

- Multiple emergencies

- Difficult patient or relative while patient deteriorating

- Criticism during emergencies

- Inadequate training during emergencies

- Unexpected complications during procedure

- Treatment started empirically before diagnosis confirmed

Remember to try to select examples ***relevant to surgery*** to demonstrate your skills and attributes to the selectors whenever answering questions on the application form and at interview. Surgeons are generally not interested in hearing about the management of chronic medical/psychiatric conditions, even if the example demonstrates your ability to make sound judgement under pressure!

Sample response

[Situation]

Whilst on-call I admitted a patient with acute pancreatitis. I sent all relevant routine investigations to complete a severity assessment.

[Problem]

Before the results were available, I noticed that the patient had become dyspnoeic. I thus prioritized the remainder of the assessment and focused on getting the arterial blood gas analysis results. These revealed that he was in type I respiratory failure.

[Action]

As the rest of my team were in the operating theatre with a laparotomy, I referred directly to the high dependency unit. I commenced resuscitation concentrating on his breathing and circulation. The rest of the blood investigations revealed failure of 2 other systems. Accordingly, he was transferred to the high dependency unit where aggressive monitoring and tailored therapy were commenced.

[Outcome]

By the time my seniors had finished in theatre the patient's respiratory exchange had normalized with non-invasive ventilation. He also had a reasonable urine output despite evidence of a raised serum creatinine. The patient spent 4 days in HDU but otherwise made an uneventful recovery. I learned the importance of sound clinical judgement and not deferring appropriate management based on such observations.

Summary

To be competitive for entry into surgical training you need to demonstrate the following key qualities, attributes and skills of a surgeon:

- Decisive thinking

- Cool head under pressure

- Awareness of own limitations

- Obsessive attention to detail

- Organized, methodical and logical

- Mentorship and leadership skills

- Good communicator

- Healthy paranoia to increase vigilance for perioperative complications

- Technical competence

- Comprehensive understanding of total body anatomy and physiology

- Conversant with management of critically sick patients

When answering clinical questions, use the **six As** approach to ensure that you address all the major points that your selectors are after:

- **A**cknowledge the main issue

- **A**lternative explanations taken into consideration

- **A**ttention to detail

- **A**pproach – structured

- **A**ppropriate clinical options

- **A**nticipate difficulties

20 Acute care common stem

Luke Moore

 Outline your clinical experience of particular use in this post.

Sample response

My diverse clinical experience acquired during my 2 year teaching hospital Foundation Rotation has allowed me to develop skills in practical and analytical aspects of medicine, as evidenced by my positive workplace-based assessments. In particular my A&E, acute medicine and ICU firms provided invaluable experience in assessing and managing acute medical and surgical presentations. Over and above the normal responsibilities of these posts, this included participation in the Resuscitation team, assessments made with the Critical Care Outreach team and work with the Pre-Hospital Care team. This developed not only my clinical assessment skills but enhanced my interpretative abilities with ECGs, diagnostic imaging and clinical laboratory investigations.

I also achieved certified competence at various acute practical procedures including amongst others: central venous access, lumbar puncture, nerve blocks, paracentesis, chest drain insertion and bone marrow aspiration.

My diverse Foundation rotation demanded a thorough understanding of pathophysiology and appropriate liaison with multiple specialties

The knowledge and effective communication skills I developed during these firms will continue to be vital within Acute Care. I have also sought to advance my sound core knowledge by taking and passing the MRCP Part I examination and through courses on Emergency Radiology, Emergency Cardiology, and a Practical Introduction to Intensive Care. In addition to this, I am a certified ALS provider and have been invited to undertake the Instructors course.

 What plan have you followed to develop your understanding of this specialty? How have your actions developed your insight into this specialty?

Sample response

In consideration of the diverse nature of ACCS, I have specifically planned my career thus far to achieve a broad knowledge and skill base.

During my FY1 rotation, I expressly chose a rotation incorporating intensive care and acute medicine to develop my abilities in assessing and managing critically unwell patients – vital to a continuing career in Acute Care. I have elected to spend time working within the multi-disciplinary critical care outreach team, an opportunity which allowed not only progression of my clinical skills in the acute setting but also development of my decision making processes. I further developed these skills by early on organising to sit the ALERT and later ALS courses.

To consolidate these professional developments, I selected an FY2 rotation including both emergency medicine, providing excellent insight into acute and hyper-acute situations, and renal medicine to complement my prior intensive care experience. To develop my insight into the other main component of Acute Care – anaesthesia – I arranged a taster week in this specialty. During this time I both started to gain a practical feel for the specialty and also to develop my insight into this specialty through discussion with my seniors. In addition to this, during my FY2 rotation I also presented a piece of work I conducted at a departmental audit meeting on the impact of the Outreach team and am currently in the midst of developing a small research protocol with an anaesthetic Professor on the subject of induction agents in COPD.

Communication skills

Communication and interpersonal skills. In the space below give a recent example which illustrates that you possess these skills.

Sample response

> I was recently involved in the care of a non-English speaking woman with sinister upper-gastrointestinal symptoms. I organized a professional advocate to assist me and had a detailed discussion with the patient, obtaining a clear picture of the clinical problem and the patient's health beliefs. By listening and appreciating these beliefs, the patient and I agreed to proceed to endoscopy with fully informed consent.
>
> I was, however, later confronted by the patient's sons who were aggressively refusing to let their mother have the procedure. In a non-confrontational manner using open body language, I defused the situation and suggested a private conversation in a side room. After first obtaining the patient's consent to discuss her medical care, I conducted a consultation with the patient's sons. Through listening, empathising with their concerns and reiterating important messages I was able to bring the whole family to concordance with the planned procedure.

Organization skills

You must be able to determine priorities and to organize your time appropriately. You will need to take responsibility for producing results with the determination to see things through to a high standard. Give a recent example that demonstrates this.

Sample response

During a recent acute medicine on call, I noticed that a patient on the admissions unit had deteriorated acutely, becoming severely agitated. I noted a new disseminated herpetic rash, and knowing the patient's immunosuppressed status, I made a clinical judgement that this was likely to represent a central nervous system infective process. Examination was limited by the patient's agitation, and as he became increasingly aggressive and a danger to others, I used appropriate sedation to make the situation safe to proceed. Acknowledging the need for quick, efficient management, I organised the necessary interventions. I arranged an anaesthetist to manage the airway prior to further sedation, the radiology team to perform urgent CT scanning and nursing colleagues to administer empirical antimicrobials whilst I performed a lumbar puncture. I then managed the patient in a level two care setting, resulting in a good recovery from viral encephalitis.

21 Paediatrics

Beverley Almeida and Elizabeth A Owen

Introduction

Paediatrics is a large and diverse specialty that attracts people for a number of different reasons. The strongest application will make clear the commitment to the specialty and have good insight into the specific skills and attributes required to be an excellent paediatrician. The application that will stand out is one that shows an applicant who is endeavouring to acquire and demonstrate these skills from an early stage; even if paediatric training has not formed part of Foundation training.

This chapter covers the following areas:

- Commitment to paediatrics
- Communication skills
- Child protection issues
- Multidisciplinary team and teamwork
- Clinical skills.

Commitment to paediatrics

Why are you motivated to pursue further training in paediatrics? In what way are you able to demonstrate that your own skills and attributes are suitable for a higher career in this specialty?

Provide evidence of your recent efforts to increase your insight and capabilities relevant to paediatrics. What has been the outcome and how has this further developed your suitability for this speciality?

You should try to demonstrate the following understanding/ skills that are demanded by a career in paediatrics when providing your response:

- Appreciation of the diverse nature of work, covering every stage from premature birth to adolescence

- Necessity to identify and manage a sick child, with special reference to not increasing problems by adding fear

- Need for good communication skills at many levels; patients of all ages, parents and families and wider agencies

- Child protection responsibilities

- Necessity for knowledge of ethics and law, especially consent, rising autonomy and refusal of treatment

- Dexterity for practical intensive procedures, such as long lines and intubation

Communication skills

Communication forms a large part of paediatrics. It is not enough to say that you communicated 'on the child's level'. You should provide specific examples that demonstrate your skills and were reflected upon.

Describe a time when you had to communicate with a child and a parent/carer in the same consultation. What approach did you take to ensure that both parties understood the issues you were discussing and how do you know if you were successful?

Sample response

In Paediatric A+E, I saw a 14-year-old with his mother (a pharmacist), attending with a first presentation of early diabetic ketoacidosis.

Once on the ward and stabilized, I explained the diagnosis to them both and educated them about the condition, under the observation of my registrar who completed a mini-CEX assessment.

The patient needed a simplistic approach but a detailed explanation. I ascertained his current understanding, he volunteered his knowledge from GCSE biology work, and I explained using similar terms, aided by simple diagrams and answering his questions. Success was indicated by checking-back his understanding.

His mother had some level of understanding of diabetes, so I spoke to her on a professional level, striking a balance between medical and lay terms, taking into account that she was upset and thus more emotional than usual. I gave them both written information to keep, and made myself available to answer further questions later.

The diabetic nurse-specialist approached me the following day informing me they both showed good understanding. His mother thanked me for being clear. The mini-CEX feedback and discussion with the registrar helped me to think about employing techniques that could be applied again in a similar situation.

To convey your communication skills relevant to paediatrics demonstrate use of:

- A traditional verbal explanation
- Pictures and diagrams
- Simple models to make it playful
- Leaflets that can be taken away
- Ability to tailor to the level of understanding of the child (e.g. younger children may respond to a practical demonstration on a toy)
- Empathy whilst imparting information and willingness to return for further explanation
- Reflection from those involved to ensure adequate understanding

Other questions that have been asked during recent application processes include:

Describe a time when you had to communicate with a young adult and a parent/carer about treatment options. What techniques did you use and what was the outcome?

Describe a time when your communication skills helped a young person and parent/carer to make a difficult decision about treatment. What approach did you take, what was the outcome and how has it informed your subsequent practice?

Child protection issues

Paediatricians have an absolute responsibility to issues of child protection – at every level of training. The safety and welfare of children is paramount. As an advocate for your patient, you have a duty to speak up and, following the Laming report, you are responsible for sharing your concerns with senior colleagues. Questions on this topic are more likely to present at the interview stage but could reasonably be posed on the application form. You would not be expected to have managed a complicated child protection case alone. However, you must demonstrate a good understanding of what is expected of a junior trainee and how to approach suspicious situations. Often a longer word count would be given – reflecting the complexity of issues involved. A formal requirement of paediatric training now involves child protection teaching and courses; make sure that this is reflected on your application form.

Describe a time when you were worried about the safety of a child. What did you do and how did you broach this with the parents/carers?

Sample response

A 3-year-old child presented with her mother who had found blood in her underwear. I took a thorough history including any suggestion of injury, unsupervised play or contact with other people, not forgetting medical concerns such as constipation or any other bleeding.

When I took a social history, her mother revealed that they lived in a small women's refuge following domestic violence, although she initially failed to volunteer this. The child had been playing alone with an 11-year-old boy that day. I explained to her mother my concerns and the need for senior involvement. Having established trust with the child and mother, I undertook a full external examination, asking the registrar to be present. There was no evidence of external injury. Our consultant was contacted and the child admitted to the ward with her mother. She was relieved to have her previously unstated concerns taken seriously and was happy to co-operate. Although a medical cause for presentation was established, this case highlighted to me many important aspects of dealing with sensitive and suspicious circumstances.

The above example highlights the difficulties of being succinct and avoiding unnecessary wordy explanations, especially when setting the scene. The response also demonstrates a good understanding of how to approach a child in possible danger. Open communication, honesty and the taking of a thorough history are important, while escalation to senior level is essential. In addition, it shows continued involvement for self-learning purposes. In the reflection section, it would have been better to expand on more specific examples of what had been learnt from the situation.

For child protection questions:

- Act in the best interest of the child, put their safety first. Make this clear to the parents or carers from the start.

- Explain that you are acting in the interest of the child, e.g. 'I am helping to keep your child safe', which implies working together.

- Take a thorough and detailed history and examine the whole child.

- Complete a diagram or use the paediatric map to show injuries.

- Take a detailed social history. Don't be embarrassed to ask questions such as who else lives in their house, whether they are known to social services, etc. Map out the family tree no matter how complicated.

- Don't attribute blame.

- Always get senior involvement at an early stage.

- Be honest with the parents about your concerns and which other agencies will be contacted or involved.

Describe a time when you felt a child was in danger but the parents/carers were unwilling to cooperate. How did you overcome this and what was the final outcome?

Multidisciplinary team and teamwork

As with each specialty, teamwork and participation in multidisciplinary teams are crucial to paediatrics. Thus, you can expect this aspect to be evaluated during the application process. It is important to avoid examples that are part of your normal job or too complicated. Avoid using 'multidisciplinary team' as a buzzword but expand on the roles of different team members and reflect on what has been learnt.

Here is a good example of how to answer this type of question.

Describe a recent time when you have worked as part of a multidisciplinary team in a challenging paediatric situation. What approach did you take and how did your behaviour enable the team to achieve their objectives?

Sample response

A 9-year-old with recently diagnosed lymphoma was having great difficulty maintaining his appetite and was refusing food and medication. The family was struggling to cope at home and he was admitted to the ward.

I met the dietician informally on frequent occasions and observed the difficulty she was having. I relayed this information to the medical team. I listened to the concerns of the ward nurses who were having problems negotiating each meal and involved the play-specialist to co-ordinate reward systems. I spoke with the child and parents, trying to expand on the issues, and took initiative to discuss with the nurses and doctors of the tertiary centre, where he received chemotherapy, about the family dynamic whilst there and organized family counselling through them.

My role in his management was to co-ordinate services available to him and his family. Although this was not a formal multidisciplinary team, I learnt negotiation skills and by ensuring the team worked smoothly together with full communication felt that each member, including the family, could feel their role, efforts and frustrations appreciated.

The key to any multidisciplinary team meeting being effective is:

- Everyone has something to add from their own unique viewpoint
- Each person should have a chance to speak
- Everyone's opinion is valued and should be respected
- There is an element of compromise and negotiation to arrive at the final goal for the patient
- Delegation of work generated from the meeting

Clinical skills

As described in Chapter 17, the interview in paediatrics mirrors that of most other specialties, comprising three separate stations encompassing clinical questions, questions on academic factors (i.e. curriculum vitae/application) and questions on NHS issues (e.g. clinical governance). For the remainder of this chapter we concentrate on how to answer clinical questions, with the assistance of worked examples:

Example 1

You are in A&E with a 3-year-old boy with wheezing and difficulty breathing. His parents are distressed and unable to give a history. What is your approach?

'*I would begin by introducing myself to the child and his parents. I would then immediately assess the child and initiating simultaneous resuscitation. Rapid assessment of his airway is the most important consideration. Is he maintaining his own airway? The child should be assessed in his comfortable position, i.e. not removed from his mother's lap, in an appropriate area. I would speak calmly to the parents to let me look at him first and then we can talk about what's happening.*'

He is crying intermittently and moaning to his mother.

'*Whilst speaking gently to the child and parents, I would assess his breathing. His colour, respiratory rate (matched to age), work of breathing (nasal flare, intercostal or subcostal recession) and if possible his saturations. I would ask mother to hold some oxygen near to him if it was necessary. I would listen to his chest and assess his circulation. If they were ready to speak I would take a focused history, especially asking for any possibility of foreign body inhalation, events leading up to the present situation or previous episodes or allergy/atopy. I would initiate treatment such as bronchodilators.*'

With oxygen and salbutamol the child settles and you are clinically less worried about him; the parents are still very distressed.

'*I would then address the parents and try to alleviate their fears, offering some reassurance that he is in the right place and has made some improvement. If the parents were then more settled and could communicate effectively, I would proceed to obtain a thorough history succinctly, with particular reference to the onset and duration of the symptoms and any pre-existing illness or medications. Family and social history are important. I would proceed to a more thorough examination. I would then convey my findings to the parents and with their consent proceed to any further treatment and admit their son to the ward if necessary.'*

Example 2

You are referred a 5-month-old boy not moving his leg who is found to have a fractured femur on his X-ray. You also notice multiple unusual bruises. What do you do next?

'*I would undertake a full initial assessment with resuscitative measures as necessary. If he is otherwise stable I would instigate treatment for his fracture, including pain relief and immobilization.*

I would ask his parents for a thorough history, in relation to how long he has been like this, whether he has sustained any injuries or trauma, whether he has complained of pain or displayed any other unusual or out of character behaviour. I would take a thorough social history, asking which other relatives or adults he had regular contact with and what activities he was involved with. I would check if they had noted the bruises and if they were aware of any other marks. I would ask for the possible explanation of these. I would complete a full examination of the child, paying attention to hygiene and looking for evidence of other injuries. I would assess for signs of hepatosplenomegaly'.

What is your main differential diagnosis at this point?

'*Non-accidental injury is high on the list, but also organic cause for fracture and bruising should be considered – such as haematological or oncological – although this may be rare in this age group.'*

Considering a diagnosis of possible non-accidental injury what would you look for and what would you do?

'*I would speak to my senior colleague and check that they are happy for me to proceed and also to request that they provide a review.*

I would try to be open and honest with his parents, explaining the presence of the fracture and that it is very unusual for children who are not weight-bearing to sustain fractures themselves so this injury is possible to have been non-accidental.

I would explain that I was not attributing blame to them, but hoped that as parents they would understand that my responsibilities were towards their child and that my aim would be to keep their child safe, working with them. This would ultimately mean that we admitted their child and used the ward as a place of safety in the short term, while further investigation took place.

I would complete a paediatric map and make sure my notes were full and complete. As part of this other agencies, such as social services, should be contacted to ascertain if the family is known. Potentially the police could be involved.'

What would you do if they wanted to take the child from the ward?

'I would attempt to explain that this was not possible, for reasons of the child's health, and involve senior support. If they were still insisting or physically removing the child I would let them know that the police could and would be involved, escalating to this if necessary.'

Example 3

A 4-day-old baby is brought back to hospital with a bilirubin level of 500. What tests will you send, what treatment will you start and how will you explain this to the parents?

'This is a medical emergency and I would arrange admission to the neonatal unit for treatment – phototherapy plus likely exchange blood transfusion.

I would introduce myself to the parents, taking a history and examining the baby. I would explain to the parents the need for admission, treatment and investigations, asking permission to take these blood tests.

I would secure venous access and send the following investigations:

Full blood count – for evidence of haemolysis, also a film, requesting sample saved.

A blood group and direct Coombe's test – evidence of rhesus or ABO incompatibility, also requesting blood for partial or full exchange.

Urea and electrolytes – especially for sodium as evidence of dehydration.

Liver function tests to confirm bilirubin, including a conjugated fraction.

Glucose, in case of hypoglycaemia and therefore the need to give additional dextrose.

Urine for reducing substances and the suggestion of galactosaemia.

Blood culture and inflammatory markers – it would be sensible to investigate for sepsis and treat empirically.

I would start triple phototherapy and contact my senior to inform them of the admission and likely transfusion. I would attempt to establish central venous access via the umbilical cord – which may still be possible at 4 days of age.'

His mother has been breastfeeding and wants to continue – what would you say to her?

'I would advise that the baby may require intravenous fluids to address potential dehydration and also I would ask her mother to express milk that we would use via the nasogastric tube until we were able to allow her to breastfeed again. I would explain to her parents that sometimes babies become jaundiced and that it is relatively common to occur at this age, but this is very high and there are important causes that need to be ruled out and hence why we are investigating. I would say that I realized that this was a lot to take in, check if they had any immediate questions and make myself available if they wanted to speak to me later as well.'

22 Obstetrics and gynaecology

Rachel Nicholson

Introduction

At specialty training year 1 (ST1) level, most questions will be non-specific, looking for evidence of generic skills, such as a sound general clinical knowledge base, conscientiousness, teamworking (especially across other health-care professions), etc. However, successful candidates will be awarded marks for demonstrating an effort to show commitment to the specialty, including while at medical school. A women's health module during Foundation years is not an essential criterion for shortlisting, but would obviously be advantageous. If completion of this module is not possible, arranging extracurricular obstetrics/gynaecology experience would help identify you as an enthusiastic candidate.

Commitment to a career in obstetrics and gynaecology (O&G)

 How will this training programme and your previous training and experience help you meet your career objectives? What are your reasons for applying to this training programme?

Sample response

My career objective is to become a consultant in obstetrics and gynaecology. I thoroughly enjoyed my attachment to the specialty during medical school and especially enjoyed completing my deliveries. I also covered reproduction during my intercalated degree in physiology and did an obstetric student elective. As a result I was keen to experience a women's health module during my foundation training. During this attachment I saw a wide range of both obstetrics and gynaecology, but particularly enjoyed obstetrics. I completed an audit concerning the management of post-partum haemorrhage and helped develop a flow chart to keep in the emergency box so that it will be easier to follow the correct protocol. Now that I am coming to the end of my foundation training I feel that I have a broad range of skills that will enable me to start specialty training. This training programme will enable me to become a specialist in obstetrics and gynaecology. I hope to sub-specialise in obstetrics.

Analysis

This response could be improved by detailing the candidate's achievements at each stage of his/her career. Further, there needs to be more reflection and insight into the benefits gained from each experience. The overall impression is of a candidate who has enjoyed obstetrics and gynaecology but can't follow instructions and perhaps isn't particularly proactive.

Improved response

My interest in training in obstetrics and gynaecology developed as an undergraduate studying for an intercalated degree in physiology. I gained a sound knowledge of reproductive mechanisms and developed insight into infertility treatment. I wished to expand my exposure to obstetrics and gynaecology as a clinical student and arranged an elective in the delivery unit of a Ugandan hospital. I completed a project comparing women's attitudes to labour pain in the UK and

Uganda. During my foundation years, I have developed greater understanding of the management of gynaecological conditions and antenatal care while enhancing my clinical skills. I completed an audit of the management of post-partum haemorrhage and acted on the findings. This training programme will enable me to fulfil my plans to complete specialty training in obstetrics and gynaecology and provides the flexibility for me to pursue my interest in reproductive and obstetric medicine. (250 words)

Having reviewed the job description and person specification, you should use this section of the form to make a statement about your career intentions and to provide additional information to support your application. This may include special interests, more detail about research, audits, publications, whether or not you have acted up on a registrar on-call rota, etc., and your leisure activities away from work. (400 words maximum)

This is a generous word allowance, but should be used wisely as this question covers a tremendous amount. You are invited to make a statement about yourself so you should start by making an impact.

'I am a motivated junior doctor with the intention of becoming a specialist obstetrician.' This is more interesting and more positive than *'I hope to become a consultant in obstetrics'*.

You should structure your response by covering the following areas:

- Career statement
- Specialist interests and achievements (within O&G)
- Interests outside of O&G (and why this makes you a better candidate)
- Leadership/management (as a doctor or outside medicine)
- Teaching (including non-medical)
- Community services (any)
- IT skills

Clinical skills

*Please give details of your clinical experience and level of competence. Do **not** list numbers of specific procedures. If you were to be appointed, what would your training priorities be for the next 12-month post?*

This question is two-part so ensure both parts are answered. Let's consider a sample response to the first part.

Sample response

I have a broad experience of different medical and surgical specialties and have ensured that my logbook is kept up to date throughout my foundation training. I am competent in managing ward patients including recognising and initiating treatment of post-operative problems. I am able to assess emergency admissions and instigate investigations and appropriate treatment. Although confident in my training and the skills that I have gained thus far, I know the limitations of my capabilities and when to seek senior help and advice. I am able to prioritise tasks when busy and I am happy managing the first on call 'take' in all the specialties I have worked in.

Nobody wants a junior incapable of making a decision; neither do they want to employ someone who will make decisions beyond their capabilities. By mentioning a logbook you have shown that you can practise clinical governance and have also given interviewers something to ask about. You have also shown that you are safe by acknowledging your limitations. If you have taken the time to try and acquire a skill that most of your peers won't have, then be sure to include it in your response (e.g. attendance at ultrasound sessions or colposcopy clinics). Applicants from Foundation training will have a record (DOPS) of their procedural experience. This should make it easy to demonstrate that you have acquired certain skills.

The second part gives you the opportunity to show that you can manage your own training and have a sensible short-term plan to fit in with your long-term goals. You should have clear objectives. Here is a sample response:

'I anticipate gaining the first part of MRCOG.' 'I plan to attend the (XXX) course on the management of obstetric emergencies.' As well as aiming to build on your previous experience and develop your abilities to manage the delivery suite/gain experience in practical skills, etc. Again you can draw attention to the skills you have, but identify any deficiencies with your training thus far, with your plans of how you will try and rectify this over the next year.

Try to demonstrate drive, enthusiasm and initiative in your answers. You must demonstrate your reasons for wanting to pursue a career in O&G to the selectors and show them that you possess the necessary attributes.

Communication skills

How do you cope with a difficult colleague?

How would you break bad news to a patient?

What would you do if a colleague persistently lets the rest of the team down?

Questions relating to communication skills are commonly encountered, particularly at the interview. The scenarios may take the form of a role-play or a discussion with patients and/or other professionals.

If you are talking to a 'patient' don't use jargon, or long-winded explanations, and make sure that the 'patient' has understood what you have said. Get a senior colleague to help. If you are worried about your communication skills, practise scenarios with your friends and family – non-medics will be able to tell you if you are easy to understand from a patient's perspective!

Please describe a situation where communication didn't go well and explain what you would do differently in the future.

Sample response

I got upset with a ward nurse because I thought I had asked her to check a patient's observations hourly and let me know if the urine output was continuing to fall. She hadn't checked and so I was unsure as to how much fluid my patient needed. However when we discussed things further I realized that I hadn't made myself clear or explained why I was worried about the patient. I now ensure that I explain my requests properly and document them in the patient's notes in order to minimize confusion. I also work hard to control my emotions with my colleagues as conflict is unlikely to be productive.

Reflective practice may also be brought into the clinical skills section. It is worth thinking about an example from your clinical practice thus far that you can talk about. Don't have anything complicated to discuss, just a simple lesson such as double-checking an investigation is enough to show that you have learnt from your experience.

Summary advice:

- Know your portfolio
- Think about answers to questions that you are likely to be asked (including 'Why do you want to do O&G?')
- If you struggle with role-play, practise with friends
- Above all, be utterly truthful in your answers
- Relax, smile and show your enthusiasm for the specialty

23 Radiology

Shilpa Patel

Questions that appear on the radiology application form tend to be generic in nature, but some have a radiological spin. It is important to answer the questions with commitment to radiology in mind.

Skill areas for potential radiologists

- Communication: Not only in discussing requests with clinicians and colleagues, but also in presenting at multidisciplinary team (MDT) meetings and written communication in radiology reports.

- Observation: This is the key in this specialty: the ability to distinguish abnormal from normal. This is a skill that can be developed.

- Dexterity: Important for the practical aspects of radiology.

- Knowledge: Particularly of anatomy and pathology.

Commitment to radiology

Why are you motivated to pursue a career in this specialty? In what way are you able to demonstrate that your own skills and attributes are suitable for a career in this specialty?

Poor example

I have been interested in a career in radiology for a very long time. It is a very important specialty and the radiologist is an essential member of the clinical team, upon whose opinion, important clinical decisions are made. The work will be varied with multiple subspecialties in which I could later specialize.

I have always enjoyed anatomy and pathology, which is very important in radiology. I completed an anatomy intercalated BSc during medical school. I have excellent problem-solving skills and am a very good observer. It is important to communicate well with all members of the multidisciplinary team, and I have proven that this is one of my strengths both at work and outside.

Better response

Radiology interests me because it is a varied subject impacting on many other clinical specialties. Whilst working closely with clinical radiologists, I have been fascinated by the range of technologies available to image the human body. I find the visual aspects of the work absorbing and the logical approach appeals to my analytical mind. This rapidly advancing field presents numerous areas to specialize in and exciting opportunities for research.

At medical school, I received a certificate of high commendation in anatomy and pathology, providing a solid basis for the academic side of radiology. Strong scores in my DOPS assessments demonstrate high levels of dexterity; my excellent references and mini-PAT assessments prove that I work well within a multidisciplinary team. My creative artwork exhibits my hand–eye co-ordination skills and my observational skills are evidenced by my ability to quickly grasp difficult routines at my weekly salsa dancing classes.

Provide evidence of activities/achievements over and above your regular scheduled daily activities that demonstrate your personal commitment to the specialty (or development of relevant skills). Indicate date and place relating to the evidence.

The key statement is *'over and above'* your duties. Therefore, do *not* simply list the daily duties of your job, even those that involve the radiology department!

Poor response

I regularly attend and present at the multidisciplinary team meetings, which gives me an opportunity to review our patients' interesting radiology. I attend the radiology lunchtime SHO teaching session. I participate by taking my interesting films for discussion with my colleagues. I have observed ultrasound-guided liver biopsies of my patients. I have attended radiology-based courses, which has enabled me to become a more competent doctor. I am doing a radiology-based audit on ultrasound-guided liver biopsies. A special study module in this subject gave me an insight into the level of observational skills required. I am currently studying towards my FRCR Part 1.

Better response

Within 2 years of qualification (2006), I have passed my MRCP Part 1 & 2. I am currently working towards my final part and I aim to complete my MRCP by summer 2007. This will provide a solid academic foundation. Thereafter I intend to sit FRCR examinations.

To consolidate my learning, I attended an A&E Trauma Radiology course at Northwick Park Hospital (Dec 2006).

I initiated and completed an audit of ultrasound-guided liver biopsies at Newham University Hospital, compared to the latest British Society of Gastroenterology (BSG) guidelines (Nov 2006). This was presented as a poster presentation entitled: 'Are multiple core biopsies required to obtain an adequate diagnostic sample on ultrasound-guided liver biopsies?' (Lisbon Medical Conference, 2007).

To improve my hand–eye co-ordination skills, I have observed and assisted in more than 10 ultrasound-guided liver biopsies (June–Sept 2006). I have registered with The Society of Radiologists in Training (2006).

They have asked for specific dates, so make sure you remember to include these. The second example demonstrates better the desired qualifications, initiative and evidence of audit, all of which are in the job description.

Interview questions

In addition to generic questions (see Chapter 17), you will clearly be asked questions specific to radiology.

Typical examples of topics/questions encountered in radiology interviews:

- *Teleradiology/outsourcing.*
- *The capabilities/limitations of the radiology department.*
- *Describe a barium enema to a patient.*
- *How has your training so far prepared you for a career in radiology?*
- *Should there be 24-7 radiology service?*
- *What qualities do you have to be a good radiologist?*
- *What do you know about the national breast screening programme?*
- *What Information Technology (IT) experience do you have?*
- *How will knowledge of IT be helpful in radiology in the next few years?*
- *Role of the radiologist in MDT meetings.*
- *Advantages and disadvantages of PACS.*

Where do you see radiology in the next 10 years?

Q: *What are the key considerations when answering this question?*

A: These can be categorized as follows:

Service level

- There will be increased numbers of radiologists but demands will also be greater, as clinicians are relying more on radiological investigations before planning management.

- Skills mix will be more streamlined to provide a service, with radiographers trained to do a variety of procedures.

- All hospitals may have well-established filmless systems, which has far reaching implications. The most obvious and beneficial is instant access to patients' imaging records from anywhere there is a terminal, whether within the hospital or outside, e.g. GP practices, other hospitals and globally.

Clinical and imaging level

- Faster and more streamlined CT and MRI scanners coupled with more flexible software investigations such as MR angiograms, virtual colonoscopies and bronchoscopies will be more readily available and routine.

- Functional imaging such as PET and SPECT will become more widely available and will play a larger role in planning a patient's management.

- Digital imaging is now replacing films and cassettes, thus providing greater accuracy in obtaining images.

Other implications:

- As services expand, screening will be important, e.g. breast cancer, colorectal cancer.

- We have a responsibility in regulating the levels of exposure of radiation to a patient.

- There will be inevitable cost implications.

Do you agree with radiographers having an extended role?

Q: *What are the key considerations when answering this question?*

A: These can be categorized as follows:

- The patient should not be exposed to unreasonable risk

- The person who undertakes the task should have undergone the necessary training

- A clinical radiologist who remains fully responsible for all aspects of the work delivered should monitor the scheme. However, the degree of supervision should not be so great that delegation is considered superfluous

- Written protocols representing departmental policies should be in place

Advantages:

- Radiographers may gain greater job satisfaction

- Radiologists will have more time to devote to activities that better match their level of expertise

- Government targets (i.e. waiting times, etc.) will be more easily achievable

Disadvantages:

- De-skilling of radiologists is a potential risk

- Inadequately defined lines of responsibility

24 Psychiatry

David Middleton

Introduction

To become a successful psychiatrist, a number of key skills are required. The selectors will be looking for trainees who are both capable and safe. The application form and interview will give you the opportunity to demonstrate the key skills necessary for a career in psychiatry.

Key attributes/skills you need to demonstrate to the selectors:

- **Excellent communication skills.** This is particularly important in a specialty where few conventional tests are available and the most essential information is often obtained from and shared with the patient, their family and other professionals.

- **Ability to work in a multidisciplinary team.** This is becoming increasingly important to the psychiatrist as more members of the team are taking on traditionally doctor-only roles. You may be asked how you would deal with such changes and how you see your role in such teams.

- **Risk assessment.** In psychiatry, you will often be treating patients who pose a risk to themselves and/or others. Make sure you demonstrate that you have considered this aspect in any scenario you are presented with. Your future consultants on the panel will want a 'safe' trainee under their tutorship.

- **Problem-solving.** More so than in many other specialties, psychiatry requires flexible thinking and an ability to decide on solutions where conventional treatment and management are not appropriate.

- **Coping under pressure.** Having an awareness of how you would cope when you have high-risk or seriously ill patients under your care will demonstrate that you have considered the more challenging aspects of the specialty.

Try thinking about how you would answer each of the following questions, remembering to tailor your response to *your* strengths.

Commitment to psychiatry

Provide evidence of your recent efforts to increase your insight and capabilities relevant to psychiatry. What has been the outcome and how has this further developed your suitability for psychiatry?

Poor response

It is good to keep up-to-date with knowledge and skills. I am going to sit the Membership of the Royal College of Psychiatrists Paper 1 exam again in March and hope to become a member of the Royal College of Psychiatrists soon. I attend the medical staff committee, risk management forum and Foundation Trust Working Group. They have all helped me with my communication skills. I have done voluntary work for the mental health charity, Mind, and have raised £1000 by completing a fun run recently. I subscribe to the Psychiatric Bulletin and British Journal of Psychiatry.

Good response

> *I understand the importance of psychiatrists maintaining both their clinical and professional skills. I have attended an exam preparation course and am sitting the MRCPsych Paper 1 in March. I am currently a Pre-Membership Psychiatric Trainee of the Royal College of Psychiatrists. As the local Paper 1 trainee representative, I have attended MMC conferences which directly led to the Specialist Training Pilot in our area. My communication skills have improved by representing peers in the medical staff committee meetings and disseminating information from this to colleagues. My voluntary work for 'Mind' gives me another important perspective of mental health care. I keep abreast of local changes in psychiatry as an active committee member of the Foundation Trust Working Group and am helping to prepare the application for Foundation Trust status. I am the junior doctors' representative on other committees including the Risk Management Forum, enabling me to broaden my understanding of important areas in the working environment.*

When trying to demonstrate your commitment to psychiatry consider:

- Becoming involved with a mental health charity
- Becoming a Pre-Memebership Psychiatric Trainee of the Royal College of Psychiatrists and being aware of some of the College's activities (www.rcpsych.ac.uk)
- Forming a local psychiatry discussion group with like-minded trainee colleagues
- The demands of a career in psychiatry

As long as you come across as enthusiastic and can demonstrate how you have channelled this enthusiasm, you should score highly in this type of question. Other sample questions that have tested commitment to psychiatry in recent years include:

Q1: Please detail any activities over and above your regular scheduled daily activities that demonstrate your personal commitment to psychiatry and explain how these activities have given you a realistic insight into psychiatry.

Q2: Describe evidence of your clinical skills in psychiatry and areas in which you need to improve. Which area has been most challenging?

Communication skills

Describe how your ability to communicate made a significant difference to a patient or carer. What skills did you demonstrate and how did they affect the patient or carer?

Sample response

I assessed an elderly man with his daughter following a referral from his GP reporting 'failing memory'. His daughter was hostile from the start and I felt quite intimidated by her attitude. Following careful exploration of the cause of her anger, it emerged that it involved her poor understanding of her father's condition combined with the distress caused by some of his upsetting comments about his late wife.

I assessed his clinical presentation and it became clear that there was evidence of a psychotic depression in addition to the already-diagnosed dementia. I carefully explained to the daughter both conditions and their role in some of her father's derogatory comments which had upset her so much. My ability to identify the cause of the daughter's anger led to a re-assessment of diagnosis and his subsequent improvement on medication. I received written feedback from the family praising my explanation.

Analysis

Hopefully, you will be able to display your communication abilities at interview but in order to get that far you will need to first put your skills on paper. Think of a scenario where you played a key role in communicating information to a patient or colleague. It might have been a 'difficult' relative as in the above example or a patient who needed particular communication techniques to extract crucial information. You should also emphasize the impact it had on the patient's care.

Describe how you would explain schizophrenia to the family of a patient recently diagnosed with this condition.

Sample response

Schizophrenia is a mental illness which affects approximately 1% of the population. People with schizophrenia may experience unusual thoughts and hallucinations and behave in an unusual manner. In men, it is often diagnosed in the late teens or early twenties. Most people will have episodes of illness followed by periods of being well. Approximately one in five will have just one episode of illness and a minority will have ongoing symptoms. The cause of schizophrenia is not known. Schizophrenia can run in families and the chances of developing it are higher in inner city areas and in drug-users. Most people will require medication called antipsychotics to help reduce and limit some of the symptoms. These can be taken in tablet form or some people prefer an injection every few weeks. Follow-up by members of a community mental health team and at outpatient appointments will help monitor symptoms and identify any emerging problems. There is no 'cure' for schizophrenia but the support from mental health services should help manage much of the condition. I can recommend a few websites for you to get more information and then have another discussion with you next week.

Empathy and understanding

Describe an incident from your experience in psychiatry when you found it difficult to understand the concerns of a patient or relative. How did you overcome this?

Sample response

A man was admitted due to severe suicidal intent following the death of his wife. His family, who regularly attended the ward round, seemed resentful towards the staff. They continually claimed that staff and students were causing their father to deteriorate but would not explain why. I initially felt very protective of my colleagues and students. I spoke to the family after one ward round and it emerged that they believed that any discussion of suicidal ideation would increase the risk of suicide. It also became clear that the family had not grieved for their mother and some of their hostility was the displacement of these emotions. My explanation made a significant difference to the family and demonstrated that information is vital to allow full understanding of some of the areas we often assume patients and their carers will understand. The team received a thank you card when the patient was discharged.

Clinical skills

Explain how you would assess the level of risk in a 72-year-old patient who has presented to A&E with an overdose of ibuprofen and is 'medically fit' to go home.

Sample response

I would want to carry out a thorough psychiatric assessment paying particular attention to the patient's mental state, past psychiatric history and risk. The details of the overdose including perceived lethality of the method and intent, planning, final acts, precautions against being discovered and how he sought help should all be noted. It would be important to gauge the patient's feelings after the overdose and if there were any ongoing suicidal thoughts. In the mental state examination, I would look for evidence of depression, especially anhedonia and hopelessness, psychotic symptoms and any effect of alcohol or drug use. Any current social stressors should also be identified. Collateral information from a relative or another healthcare professional would help inform my assessment. Demographic risk factors such as male sex, single/divorced/widowed, poor social contact, old age or unemployment should be taken into account. The presence of specific risk factors such as substance misuse, previous suicide attempts, recent psychiatric admission or chronic medical illness would raise my concern. I would decide on whether the patient should be managed at home or in hospital and would assess his capacity and insight to determine if admission under the Mental Health Act should be considered. I would discuss any concerns I had with my senior and also try to involve the patient and his family in the decision-making process as far as possible.

Describe an example from your experience in psychiatry when applying your clinical judgement had a significant impact on a patient's care.

Sample response

Whilst on call, I was asked to assess an elderly patient who had become agitated and aggressive. I was asked to prescribe something to 'settle her down'. I had not met the patient previously but from collateral history, it was clear that this was unusual behaviour for her. A thorough physical examination revealed that the change in presentation could have been due to a cerebrovascular event so I made arrangements for a CT scan. The medical registrar felt that her symptoms were probably due to antipsychotic side effects so I had to insist on further assessment by his team. The CT scan revealed an acute-on-chronic subdural haematoma of considerable size. The patient was transferred for surgical intervention and returned a week later when she was interacting and communicating clearly for the first time in 2 years. Her family thanked me and the team for our intervention.

A 30-year-old male admitted with his first episode of mania has developed a fever, dizziness and is complaining of aching arms. He had needed medication the previous day due to aggressive behaviour but is now more confused than before. What would you suspect? How would you manage him?

Sample response

I would want to rule out neuroleptic malignant syndrome and would therefore request that the nursing staff administer no further neuroleptic medication until fully assessed. I would ask for a set of physical observations to be carried out, including lying and standing blood pressure readings. I would next carry out a full physical examination and look for the presence of increased muscle tone, hyperthermia, autonomic instability and confusion. Investigations including blood tests for FBC, U&Es and creatinine kinase should also be sent. It would also be important to consider other diagnoses such as meningitis or septicaemia. I would arrange transfer to an acute medical ward for intensive monitoring and treatment. This treatment might include intravenous fluid resuscitation, benzodiazepines for behavioural disturbance and dantrolene or bromocriptine to reduce muscle rigidity. Finally, it would require careful consideration in the future for reintroduction of neuroleptic medication and a clear documentation of the sensitivity in the patient's records.

Other sample questions that have been asked in recent years include:

What has influenced your choice of a career in psychiatry?

You receive a call from the ward nurse telling you that a 23-year-old male patient wants to leave the ward. He was transferred from the medical ward having attempted to hang himself 1 week ago. How would you deal with the situation? How and when could the Mental Health Act be used in this situation?

You are called about a female patient who was admitted to your ward 2 days ago with symptoms of depression. She has become aggressive and confused and reported seeing animals in her bed. What is your differential diagnosis and how would you manage the situation?

You visit a 75-year-old man at his home 6 weeks after the death of his wife. It is clear that he has not been eating well and his hygiene is poor. He is low in mood but does not want to come into hospital. How would you deal with the situation?

To help ensure that you secure a specialty training (ST) post in psychiatry:

- Know the common themes that present themselves on the application form and at interview

- Familiarize yourself with legal issues

- Display your tailored and specialized communication skills

- Show empathy

25 Infectious diseases and medical microbiology/ virology

Luke Moore

Introduction

Infectious diseases are one of the last bastions of acute multi-system secondary care medicine. The role of an infectious disease practitioner is primarily as a diagnostician, and dual accreditation with microbiology or virology enables the trainee to develop a broad base of skills within the field of infection.

Mention the following hot topics to help secure your specialty training (ST) post:

- Sepsis and the surviving sepsis campaign
- Tropical diseases/international health problems (the big three being TB, malaria and HIV)
- Infection control/health-care-associated illness (particularly MRSA and *Clostridium difficile*)
- Historically, infectious disease has been a very academically orientated specialty, so emphasize your achievements and aspirations in that direction as well

Commitment to specialty

Please outline your career to date and show how your experiences have contributed to your professional development and to your application for a post as ST3 in infectious diseases and medical microbiology/virology.

Poor response

My career to date has contributed to my wish for a career in Infectious Diseases and Medical Microbiology. I have undertaken several steps towards this. The first was the completion of my intercalated BSc in Microbiology within which my dissertation taught me a lot on the topic of Borreliosis. After graduating, I undertook a medical rotation, and managed to obtain my full MRCP which has contributed to my professional development. During this time I completed an audit on Clostridium difficile which was published. During my career break in 2007, I was offered a place on the Diploma of Tropical Medicine at the London School of Hygiene & Tropical Medicine which consisted of lectures, seminars and exposure to laboratory work – mainly in the form of parasitology. For my ST2 year I have been assigned a rotation including a 4-month firm in Tropical Medicine and having successfully completed both inpatient and outpatient duties. I feel I now want to pursue this as my career.

Better response

My interest in infective pathology developed during my intercalated BSc in Microbiology. From this I derived not only a strong microbial knowledge but also autonomy and practical ability in laboratory practice. During my medical rotation I quickly passed the MRCP examination and developed a greater understanding of the clinical application of infection and infection control. One of my many audits included work on Clostridium difficile, which was published in the Journal of Antimicrobial Chemotherapy. To further my postgraduate training, I obtained a place on the Diploma of Tropical Medicine, enhancing my clinical skill base and developing my interest in host–microbe interactions and diagnostics. I have obtained an ST2 post in Tropical Medicine in which I am putting my postgraduate studies in infection into practice. In addition I have organized rotating around microbiology, virology and parasitology for a session a week to expand my understanding of the practicalities of laboratory medicine.

Analysis

Both answers score in the fields of clinical governance (audit) and academia (publication). The 'well scoring' candidate expresses the learning points attained from each experience. The poorly scoring answer concentrates on the specifics of each activity, for example, naming the institution where the diploma was undertaken, rather than mentioning any transferable skills acquired.

Discuss what you think is currently the most important issue in infectious diseases and medical microbiology.

Poor response

I think that malaria is currently the most important issue in infectious diseases and medical microbiology. This is because Malaria affects lots of people worldwide and children especially are at risk of dying. Here in the UK we also get a lot of malaria patients from people who travel abroad. I have had ample experience in treating patients with malaria during my infectious disease firm and I feel confident in the management of this disease. There have been a lot of recent developments in the treatment of malaria and work is currently ongoing on a malaria vaccine. I think that the combination of vaccine and more efficient therapy will see malaria become less important as my career progresses. I wish to pursue an active role in international infectious diseases during my career, and would like to focus my future postgraduate development in the field of malaria.

Better response

Tuberculosis (TB), with an estimated 8 million new cases a year worldwide, up to 2 million deaths per year, and an increasing rate of drug resistance is perhaps the most important issue in the field of infection. TB provides many hurdles for the infectious diseases and microbiology professions to overcome. Diagnostics for this disease are slow to evolve – mainly due to pathogen specific factors, and treatment of this disease is a continuing practical issue. The emergence and rapid spread of both multi- and extended-drug resistant tuberculosis is a growing threat, and will become a greater issue for UK physicians as immigration and travel become even more omnipresent. My previous audit work on source isolation for air-borne pathogens, combined with the doctorate proposal I am initiating in the field of TB diagnostics continue to develop my knowledge, skills and enthusiasm for further work in this important field.

Analysis

The field of important issues in infectious diseases is wide, and each scorer may have their own opinion; the justification and the reflection are ultimately more important than the topic. It is still important to be well-read and knowledgeable on topical issues in the field. The international 'Big Three' are currently HIV, TB and malaria, with health-care-associated infections being very topical in the NHS.

The structure of the 'poor response' lacks cohesion – the candidate picked a suitably important topic, but did not discuss the specific impact in the field of infection. The candidate tried to impart his/her experience in this area, but this could be discussed in a more succinct and focused manner.

The better response validates the argument that TB is an important issue, and the applicant goes on to express his/her personal attributes and previous work, and provides a talking point on aspirations towards a higher degree.

- Remember who you are targeting with your answer, and tailor the emphasis accordingly

- Personalize each answer to include your experiences and skills

- Always answer the question, don't waste words by including the wording of the question in your answer

Hot topics in infectious diseases and medical microbiology

What would be the key points when putting forward a business plan for eradication of MRSA within a trust?

Q: What are the key points when addressing this question?

A: Consider:

- Use audit to establish the extent of the current problem

- Perform root cause analysis and establish areas to target interventions

- Involve the multidisciplinary team to formulate a business plan, which would then be put forward to the primary care trust

- Acknowledge that eradication may be difficult to achieve, and suppression may well be a more attainable endpoint

Intervention falls into two groups:

- Prevention: introduction of 'care bundles', use of alcogel, decreasing bed occupancy rates

- Treatment: antiseptics and topical antibiotics for colonization with use of glycopeptides for bacteraemia

- Complete the audit cycle to ascertain impact of interventions

If you were in charge of designing a new hospital which factors would you be concerned about?

Q: What are the key points when addressing this question?

A: Consider:

- The services to be provided by the hospital.
- The percentage of side rooms reflects many factors, i.e. specialist services such as renal and haematology units.
- The need for positive or negative pressure rooms will also depend on the expected patient demographics.
- Designing wards to minimize patient movement is essential, especially inter-ward transfers.
- More functional aspects of daily work must also be considered, from hygienic keyboards, to bed-end alcogel, to antibacterial uniforms.

What are the ethical and practical issues surrounding HIV testing?

Q: What are the key points when addressing this question?

A: Consider:

- Testing for HIV should still only be carried out with the consent of an individual, and after suitable pre-test counselling has occurred. More difficult consent orientated scenarios may well be presented at interview, enquiring as to one's approach to testing incompetent/obtunded individuals, and acting in best interests as well as asking for senior help are reasonable answers.
- Practically, HIV testing is currently laboratory-based in the NHS but some centres are moving towards initial testing being in the form of fourth generation 'near-patient tests' with the obligatory second (confirmatory) test occurring in the laboratory. Fourth generation tests have a high negative predictive value despite the low incidence in the UK and are therefore a reasonable first-test tool. They test for both antibody and the p-24 antigen so they can detect early HIV infections; however, there is still a window period.
- The results of tests and appropriate follow-up must also be discussed, and confidentiality must be maintained at all times.

26 Histopathology

Jane Walker

Introduction

Histopathology is a relatively small specialty with an annual intake of up to 60 trainees (the exact number is determined by workforce planning activity). Application to histopathology differs from other specialties in that it is a national process. Recruitment is only at specialty training year 1 (ST1) level, via one of the 12 schools in England and Wales (Scotland recruits separately). If you are successful in your application the job offer is for a histopathology training post, *not* for a specific school. Applicants are asked to rank their preferences for location and the places are allocated based on their performance at interview. This system improves your chances of getting a place, but means you will need to be flexible about where you are willing to work.

Before you apply for a histopathology training job it is useful to be familiar with the following websites:

- www.nhshistopathology.net – this is the training schools' website and has information about each of the training schools, details about how to apply, and also an online forum for prospective applicants

- www.rcpath.org.uk – this is the website for the Royal College of Pathologists and has information about the specialty, as well as recent advances and news articles

Commitment to specialty

Histopathology is not a specialty that you will necessarily have had much exposure to unless you have done a 4-month rotation as part of your foundation training. You are *not* expected to have worked in the department. However, you will be expected to have shown some initiative and learned as much as you can about the job.

What plan have you followed to develop your understanding of histopathology? How have your actions developed your insight into this specialty?

Sample response

I first became interested in pursuing a career in histopathology at school, when I spent time in the histopathology department at a nearby hospital before applying for medical school. I was able to observe the processing of specimens, from their arrival at the lab to the final microscopy and subsequent diagnosis. I continued to improve my understanding of histopathology at university where I organized a Special Study Module in cytology, enabling me to become a proficient microscopist, and to learn more about this aspect of a pathologist's role and its importance in the cervical screening programme. I regularly attended post mortems and was fascinated by the logical approach needed to correlate the post mortem findings with the clinical history. During my foundation training I arranged taster days in the histopathology departments of two local hospitals, consolidating my understanding of the specialty and allowing me to learn some basic immunohistochemistry.

- Apply for a foundation rotation with a pathology job in it.
- Arrange to spend some 'taster days' with a histopathologist. Try to see a little bit of all the aspects of the job so that you have an overall idea of what the job entails.

- Spend time in a histopathology laboratory – observe how the specimens are processed from their arrival in the laboratory to the final issuing of the report, and how this relates to patient care.

- If you have a surgical rotation, attend as many multidisciplinary teams (MDTs) as you can to understand the role of the pathologist in the diagnosis and treatment of disease.

- Organize and implement an audit related to pathology.

- Think back to your time at medical school – did you do any pathology-orientated Special Study Modules? Did you intercalate a degree, either in pathology or in a relevant area such as anatomy?

- Speak to existing trainees.

- Be familiar with the Royal College of Pathologists website.

- Be familiar with particularly well publicized areas such as screening programmes and the human tissue act.

The interview

The interview is designed to ensure that you have the right qualities to be a histopathologist and that you are motivated to pursue this career. Previously, it has consisted of six 5-minute face-to-face interviews that will expand on the information given on the application form. It is highly structured with strict time limits. Therefore, it is important that your answers are concise and to the point. You will also be given a chance to discuss your portfolio briefly.

There will be a short written exercise as part of the interview. This is not to test your knowledge of histopathology, but to assess your written communication. This is a generic skill, not specific to this specialty.

A colleague is considering leaving histopathology. Discuss the advantages and disadvantages of a career in this specialty.

Sample response

Histopathology is a fascinating, rapidly changing area of medicine. It plays a vital role in the diagnosis and treatment of disease. As a histopathologist you work closely with other members of the MDT to ensure the patient is given an accurate prognosis and the appropriate therapy. There are ample opportunities to become involved in teaching and research as a histopathologist and this adds to the varied nature of the job. It is also possible to manage your workload to a certain degree, and this gives greater flexibility in the working hours. There is little or no out of hours commitment meaning that it is easier to achieve a successful work-life balance than it perhaps is in other specialities.

On the negative side, there is often no patient contact and so you do not directly see the results of your work. There can be a lot of pressure to report cases promptly and meet targets and, if you are not able to manage your time effectively, the workload can pile up. Because each consultant works somewhat independently, taking any unplanned leave can lead to a backlog and further time pressures if this situation is not dealt with promptly.

You, as a consultant histopathologist, come to work one day to find that all of your consultant colleagues have phoned in sick leaving you alone with two trainees. How will you deal with this?

Sample response

I would first establish exactly what work needed doing that day. For example, are there any MDTs? Are there any post mortems? I would then look at what had to be done that day, and what could be re-scheduled. Once completed, I would assess what I would have to do myself, and what could be delegated to the trainees. I would prioritize any cases that needed reporting urgently for clinic appointments or MDTs, and any specimens that needed to be cut up urgently. If there was an MDT it would be difficult to reschedule this, but it may be that one of the trainees would be happy to go alone if I went through the slides with them first. Depending on the seniority of the trainees it is likely that they would at least be able to cut up routine specimens unsupervised, and may be able to do the post mortems and then present their findings to me, thus freeing up my time to report the urgent cases. By prioritizing the work and delegating to the trainees, I would hope that the urgent cases could be dealt with effectively, without letting the routine work pile up significantly.

In order to answer these questions you do not need an in-depth knowledge of histopathology but you do need to know the basics and be able to present them logically. In order to discuss the pressures of the job or prioritize the work you need to know exactly what a histopathologist does. It will be obvious if you haven't researched your chosen career and spent at least some time in the department.

27 Public health

Anne Swift

Introduction

Public health is about looking after the health of populations rather than individuals. The population might be a prison, the residents of an area served by a Primary Care Trust (PCT), or maybe a whole country.

Public health is a broad specialty that involves three main areas:

- Protecting health from threats such as infectious diseases and environmental hazards.

- Promoting and improving health and wellbeing.

- Improving health services on a day-to-day basis. This can involve assessing the health of the population, seeing where improvements could be made, and dreaming up creative and effective ways to make those improvements happen while ensuring that the books balance.

Public health is also unique as a speciality since medical applicants train side by side with non-medics, in a ratio of about two to one.

As future public health consultants, applicants need to demonstrate their ability to:

- Work well in teams with other professionals

- Be a skilled communicator and show leadership when required

- Evaluate and interpret the evidence relating to health care and understand the need for evidence-based decisions about how resources should be used

- Be comfortable handling data and statistics

- Understand the nature of public health practice in the UK as compared to other countries (e.g. knowing that there is no patient contact)

- Demonstrate passion and vision for a healthier population and the skills that will make the vision a reality

Specialty training in public health: selection process

Recruitment to specialty training is a nationally coordinated process with one intake (August) per year. Posts are advertised in the *BMJ* and *Health Service Journal* and on deanery websites. Applicants make a *single* application through a central electronic portal, stating deanery of first and second choice and other deaneries acceptable if pooled. If shortlisted, applicants are interviewed at the selection centre of their first choice deanery. Scores are ranked and offers made either by the first choice or through the pool.

Candidates are invited to attend a half-day assessment centre, testing numerical and verbal critical reasoning. These are written multiple-choice tests, taken under examination conditions, and are very similar to the psychometric tests widely used in industry. Numerical reasoning requires candidates to work quickly (the time pressure is intense and you are *not* expected to finish the paper) but accurately. Questions typically require interpretation of data presented in tables or diagrams, or finding percentages and proportions of figures (you are allowed a calculator). Verbal reasoning involves exercises such as choosing logical conclusions from a passage of text or spotting where assumptions have been made. The best preparation for these tests is practice. Free sample numerical and verbal reasoning tests can be found online, and books of practice tests are widely available. Brushing up on basic maths skills is also valuable preparation for the numeracy test.

Candidates who pass both tests are eligible for shortlisting, which is undertaken by scoring the application form.

The application form

Most of the questions on the application form are likely to be quite generic, so even before the forms are available it is possible (and advisable) to prepare your thoughts. Refer to Section B of this book for advice on how to complete such questions.

Commitment to public health

Why are you motivated to pursue a career in public health? In what way are you able to demonstrate that your personal skills and attributes are suitable for a career in public health?

Poor response

Public health is the science and art of preventing disease, prolonging life and promoting health through the organized efforts of society. By working at a population level rather than with individual patients, public health professionals can improve the health of vast numbers of people and therefore make a much bigger impact on health overall. I think that I will be able to help with this endeavour and that my skills will be useful in the practice of public health. I am a good communicator, and have gained many transferable skills through working as a doctor, all of which will be of benefit in my future career. I think that there are many important public health issues facing the UK and the world today, including obesity and smoking, and wider issues such as global warming and the environment, which will provide interesting and challenging work for the future.

Better response

I am passionate about improving people's lives; health is a major determinant of quality of life and I believe that major health problems such as heart disease, diabetes and obesity are most effectively tackled at population level. Rather than reactive 'fire fighting' with individual patients, I want to be part of a creative and proactive team in devising strategies for illness prevention and to empower people to improve their own health.

Health inequalities persist and widen despite improved standards of living; I want to contribute to understanding and reversing this trend.

My proven communication and motivational skills, developed through counselling training, will enable me to listen to, persuade and inform partners in this work. I have proven skills in problem solving, coping with pressure, teamworking and organization in my clinical work and my current role in research. This mix of skills will enable me to practise effectively in public health.

Analysis

The poor response wastes many words in describing and defining public health, and although this reads reasonably well it is not relevant to the question or to the applicant. There is no personalization of motivation or relevant experience. Only communication is mentioned as a specific skill; others are alluded to but not named. The answer does not hang together well, and the overall impression is of a rather disorganized and 'cut-and-paste' approach.

The 'better response' is passionate and engaging. The applicant provides a sense of the enthusiasm for the specialty. Evidence is provided for the skills described, including from sources other than daily work (the counselling course). The answer is coherent and describes why public health appeals, and what proven skills could be brought to the specialty by the applicant. Insight into the specialty is demonstrated by mentioning skills that are very important in public health, such as motivation and teamworking.

Briefly identify from your own knowledge an area where the application of research has related to the practice of public health.

Sample response

Having trained and worked in Leicester, I am aware of the area's excess cardiovascular mortality, which is related to the large South Asian population. Research has identified ethnic risk factors, present in childhood, including a tendency to central adiposity, glucose intolerance and high insulin levels. Classical risk factors show wide variability in this population and some factors (e.g. smoking) are lower than for an equivalent European population. This clearly impacts on public health strategies for primary and secondary prevention. Stop smoking advice may be less relevant while weight control through diet and exercise are probably much more important. Overall increased risk means that guidelines for treating factors such as hypertension should be adjusted for this population. NICE guidelines emphasize that secondary prevention strategies such as cardiac rehabilitation must be made available and acceptable to populations less likely to access them, including South Asians.

Analysis

This answer provides a specific example of the application of research to public health activities such as health promotion and smoking cessation. It gives evidence for this example having been drawn from the candidate's own experience, and shows awareness of the public health aspects of cardiovascular disease. Mentioning

NICE guidelines shows an awareness of broader issues and the importance of such guidance in service planning and delivery.

At the selection centre

Shortlisted applicants are invited to attend a selection centre. This consists of multiple panel interviews, possibly including a presentation (with time given to prepare on the day), a basic level critical appraisal of a scientific paper, a group exercise or an in-tray exercise.

To excel at the selection centre:

- Practise critical appraisal of published work
- Brush up on presentation skills
- Be familiar with public health-related current affairs
- Know what's involved in a public health career in the UK

You are working as a public health registrar and the local residents' association, who are concerned about the health effects of rubbish being collected only fortnightly, contacts you. How do you handle the enquiry?

Q: What do I need to cover when answering this question?

A: First do no harm – use a step-wise approach:

- Respond to the immediate enquiry. Bear in mind that you are working under supervision and that the organization you work for is likely to have a policy for dealing with enquiries from the public. If you are not confident to answer the query straightaway then let the caller know you will get back to them. Stick to what you say you will do.

- Investigate the issue. Has this already been the subject of discussion? What was the outcome? Look at the research evidence, if there is any. Talk to your seniors and to others within (and outside) the organization. Bear in mind this issue will have a lot to do with environmental health and the district council – and may be better dealt with by them.

- Organize an action: Does more work need to be done on this? Should there be a meeting or some contact between the interested parties to try to come to an understanding? Who should attend such a meeting?

- Reflect and learn.

Other questions that have been asked in recent application processes include:

What one action should the government take to make the biggest impact on public health? Why? What problems might there be with this action?

What action have you taken to develop your understanding of public health? How have these activities developed your insight into this specialty?

Please give an example from your own work of a problem and what a public health professional might make of it.

28 Academic appointments

Philip J Smith

Academic application questions

On an academic specialty training (ST) application form, you can reasonably expect to have a mix of academic questions, as well as the questions that could appear on the non-academic application forms. Below are some of the more common questions seen on academic application forms.

Please give brief details of all the research projects and/or all the relevant research experience that you have undertaken or are undertaking, including methods used. Indicate your level of involvement and your exact role in the research team.

Sample response

I have conducted two major research projects in which I have acted as lead investigator. I designed and developed the 'Diabetes Health Locus of Control' scale for children; testing the validity and test re-test reliability of the scale against an already valid generic locus of control scale. Children with diabetes were asked to complete both scales, with the scores of each scale being analysed to test the validity of the new scale.

As part of the St Elsewhere's Central Line study group I instigated an investigation into whether there was any association between central line bacteraemia and gut bacterial overgrowth, using available microbiological data on each patient.

In both projects, I worked as part of a multidisciplinary research team, collecting data and co-ordinating its analysis. The successful completion of these projects has led to two international presentations and publication in a peer-reviewed journal.

Please describe in more detail one of the research projects mentioned above.

Sample response

Whilst working at St Elsewhere's Children's Hospital, I expressed my interest in gastroenterology and was invited to be the lead researcher testing the hypothesis that pathological overgrowth of gut organisms predisposed to bacteraemia in children with central venous lines.

Using the pooled data of over 250 patients entered into the St Elsewhere's Central Line study group, I devised a proforma to collect the data, collated and analysed this, using chi squared analysis. I was supported by a team of senior researchers and clinicians. The results suggested a statistically significant relationship between overgrowth of certain pathogenic organisms and central line bacteraemia. These results supported previous research findings in animal populations, stimulating further research involving selective decontamination of the digestive tract (SDD) agents.

This study has been presented at the 25th Congress of Paediatric Surgeons in Paris in 2005 and at the British Association of Paediatric Surgeons 27th International Conference in Cardiff in 2006.

Please say why you want this particular Academic Clinical Fellowship (ACF), indicating your medium- to long-term career goals in relation to an academic career in this specialty area.

Sample response

I have always been interested in following an academic career path. I have now had the chance to undertake two research projects, which I have thoroughly enjoyed. I would now like to pursue this interest by combining my clinical specialist registrar training with some further research projects. I would like to use this time to gain some generic research skills and to identify an area of interest which I may then develop to obtain a higher degree. This would give me a greater appreciation of the impact that high quality research has on patient care. Furthermore, I am interested in developing medical education – teaching and learning are integral to being an academic doctor. I am committed to a career in academic gastroenterology and hope that this ACF post will ultimately make me an excellent candidate for a senior lecturer position in this field.

Academic interview questions

Within an academic interview, you can reasonably expect to get a mixture of clinical questions similar to other ST trainees, but also specific questions aimed at teasing out your academic credentials.

- It is worth researching the most likely areas that will come up in the interview.

- This may involve visiting research laboratories in the institutions you are applying to.

- Speak to other research fellows and ask advice from as many academics as possible. They should be able to guide you through the most likely scenarios.

- If you know which academics will be on the interview panel, visit their laboratories, and ensure you know their areas of expertise!

Before an interview a non-exhaustive list of areas that you should be familiar with includes:

- Definition and limitations of translational research (i.e. research extending from the laboratory to the bedside – problems: funding; expensive infrastructure; practical issues; ethical issues; communication issues)

- Declaration of Helsinki and the 13 principles of Good Clinical Practice (international guidelines when setting up clinical trials)

- The different phases of clinical trials (see below)

- NICE guidelines – ensure you are familiar with at least one in your specialty and know how they work in practice

- Research funding (Wellcome Trust, Medical Research Council, private companies, charitable sources)

- Areas of particular interest for you in your specialty

- Methods by which you 'keep up to date' (peer-reviewed journals; conferences; grand rounds; journal clubs; internet)

- Ethical issues in your specialty and ethical issues in research

- Clinical governance and research governance

Phases of clinical trials

- Preclinical toxicology studies on animals

- Phase I – on healthy volunteers, establishing safe dosing

- Phase II and III – randomized control trials with patients with the disease being treated looking for efficacy

- Phase IV – professional marketing and pharmacy with ongoing assessment with the yellow card scheme

Before you go into the interview, ensure you are at the very least familiar with a recent paper that has:

- Changed practice in your specialty area
- Changed your understanding of a particular specialty topic
- Interested you although not necessarily originating from your specialty area.

Some of the examples below may help you prepare and tackle questions such as this in your academic interview.

In the last 5 years, which paper have you read that has changed your practice the most?

Sample response

In my first medical post in 2004, we had a young man admitted under our team with severe bloody diarrhoea and a relapse of his ulcerative colitis (UC), despite being on all of the available medications at that time. He was not keen to have a total colectomy, but this was deemed his only remaining treatment option, and so he proceeded to surgery. Infliximab had been used with success in Crohn's disease patients, but had not been used in treatment of UC. However, Rutgeerts et al, in December 2005, published a paper in the New England Journal of Medicine (NEJM), relating to the use of Infliximab for induction and maintenance therapy in UC. The study was widely known as the ACT1 and ACT2 trials (Active Ulcerative Colitis Trials 1 and 2), both double blind randomized placebo-controlled trials which showed that patients with moderate to severe UC were significantly more likely to respond to Infliximab over those receiving placebo over a follow-up period of time, inducing remission. This study opened the door for those with UC to another possible treatment option that was previously reserved for patients with Crohn's disease only and has changed clinical practice. If this evidence had been available at the time, the young man may have escaped a colectomy. This has made me reflect on the necessity for us, as a profession, to keep breaking down the barriers of clinical research and looking for alternative solutions to current clinical problems.

Are you aware of any papers that have influenced the practice of medicine and surgery in the last year?

Sample response

As a surgical (or anaesthetic) trainee, I read with interest a paper in the Lancet in 2008 by the POISE study group, regarding the effects of extended release Metoprolol in patients undergoing non-cardiac surgery. Previous studies have shown the benefits peri-operatively of using Metoprolol on morbidity and mortality, although some smaller studies have contradicted this belief. Indeed, in my training so far, I have been aware of the widespread use of beta blockers in the peri-operative period, in an attempt to reduce the effect of the catecholamine release in surgery. The paper described a double blind randomized placebo-control trial of over 8000 non-cardiac surgery patients. The trial showed that those receiving Metoprolol had a reduced risk of myocardial infarction 30 days post operation, but an overall increased risk of death and stroke during the same period of time. Since this paper has been published, I have noted a reduction in the number of beta blockers used peri-operatively, as a direct result of this trial's finding.

Tell me about an interesting paper you have read recently in this specialty or another. Why was it interesting?

Sample response

In the New England Journal of Medicine in December 2004, Thwaites et al published a double blind randomized placebo-control trial performed in Vietnam in patients presenting with TB meningitis (TBM) with or without HIV, showing that Dexamethasone treatment alongside anti-TB medications improves survival from TBM, but probably does not improve morbidity and disability associated with this. Recently, I had a chance to put this evidence into practice when we admitted an HIV-positive patient with confusion and a reduced GCS. With lumbar puncture findings suggesting that TB meningitis was the most likely diagnosis in this immunocompromised patient, Dexamethasone was suggested by myself and agreed by the consultant to be started alongside anti-TB medications. I found this paper particularly interesting as this research clearly had a significant positive impact on this patient's overall management. The landmark paper also suggests the recommended reducing dose regimen of Dexamethasone, which is widely accepted across the world.

To prepare for the academic interview:

- Revise all the above suggested areas

- Get advice from and visit academics before the interview

- Know your publications, presentations and posters inside out – you will probably be questioned on them

SECTION E
The good, the bad and the emergency exits

29 Successful entry into specialty training: next steps

Beverley Almeida

Introduction

So, you've negotiated the application form, had your interview and now you've secured your training post. All in all, things have gone according to plan, but unfortunately there is only a short amount of time in which to sit back and relax! After the initial elation, you have to start thinking about all the assessments and examinations required of you. These assessments and feedback are central to the new style specialty training (ST) and fulfilling them means that first you keep hold of your training post and second you keep progressing on a yearly basis.

Assessments in specialty training

Assessment determines whether you are progressing, provides evidence of your achievements and ensures that you have gained the core competencies to provide better care to patients. It also enables identification of any problems you may have as soon as they arise, encouraging you to address them in a formal setting. These assessments have been further detailed in the Modernising Medical Careers' (MMC's) *Gold Guide*. If you're a specialty trainee it's your business to know and understand what these are. Your deanery will provide you with details of exactly what and how many assessments you are expected to complete and when they should be completed by. You are responsible for organizing your own assessments and finding suitable cases and colleagues to assess you. It is ill advised to leave all of your assessments to the last months of your job or even the last weeks of your job; putting the pressure on your colleagues is not a way to make yourself popular!

Final Annual Review of Competence Progress (ARCP)

At the end of each year, these documents form part of the 'virtual' ARCP. It is intended that all your online assessments and other items uploaded on your e-portfolio are viewed online by the ARCP panel. For some deaneries this may also involve submitting an up-to-date curriculum vitae (CV), your logbook of procedures, your personal development plan and trainer's reports from your educational and clinical supervisors, although most of these items can now be completed directly on the e-portfolio. The ARCP is like the old style RITA, but as yet your attendance is not compulsory and the review does not have to be done in your presence. Therefore it pays to have everything in spick and span condition, so that it is watertight, as you won't necessarily be there to explain any gaps or anything that's missing.

Postgraduate examinations and the role of the Royal Colleges

In addition to this, obviously, are the more traditional college exams. It is still vital that you pass the examinations for the college of your choice as they are a mandatory component of assessment in the UK training curriculum for all the specialties.

Previously, gaining membership to your chosen college was the normal requirement for higher ST, i.e. to progress to registrar level you had to have passed all these examinations to become a member. However, the nature of ST is that it is competency-based, not examination-based, so there now seems to be some leeway. Membership for some of the colleges is no longer essential to progress to SpR level (ST3 for most specialties).

Regardless of all of this the colleges remain important as they are responsible for the curriculum and overall the standard of your training. In addition, enrolling in your college and paying the necessary fees is now essential for most, as it provides access to your online assessments and access to your e-portfolio, which as mentioned above must all be completed to fulfil your training.

Other requirements to progress successfully through specialty training

Once you've passed your exams and completed all the required assessments you can then concentrate your time and efforts on enhancing your CV in other (more exciting and interesting) ways and re-addressing the balance between work and your social life and hobbies. Don't disregard the next step, i.e. re-application and progression from core to ST. Work on the aspects you found to be sparse or deficient during this application. The specialties that have remained run-through will not necessarily always be so.

To keep your career progressing, ensure that you:

- Complete required assessments on time

- Update your e-portfolio regularly

- Prepare for your ARCP and take it seriously

- Are successful in your college's exams

- Develop your CV for the next application

- Don't forget the ultimate goal, to become a good consultant

30 Failure to gain entry into specialty training: what next?

Zohra Ali, Chris Godeseth and Philip J Smith

When the unthinkable has happened, after all the hard work there is nothing to show for it. Somehow, somewhere along the line, something went very wrong and you are left out in the cold, without a single job offer on the table. What next? Here are a few ideas.

1. Don't panic!

You will not be the first or the last person in this situation.

2. Find employment

Understandably, the source of ongoing immediate employment is likely to be of primary concern. Aside from specialty training (ST) posts there remain numerous opportunities for employment, albeit in a non-training capacity on the whole. These include the following:

- *Gaining an extension to your current contract* – Trusts where staff members have made a good impression are often keen to retain their services, either in their current or a similar role. Bear in mind that this may not be possible due to allocation of new specialty trainees into post, but it's always worth speaking with your consultants and Human Resources.

- *Stand-alone posts* (such as Clinical Fellows or service locum posts [LAS]) are also regularly advertised, but try to be selective in what you apply for. Use this as an opportunity to build on your experience to date; perhaps explore an area that could teach you valuable skills, and be generically applied to any specialty area. ITU for example, previously formed a key element of many of the basic medical and surgical rotations of old.

- Further *specialty-specific experience* could be gained, as a taster, if your experience is limited or to further demonstrate your commitment if applying at a more senior level. At senior levels (ST3 and above), locum training posts (LAT) can be applied for independently, with the additional benefit that retrospective training credit is awarded for all time in post.

- *Research* also remains an option at all levels of training, and should especially be considered by more senior level applicants. This could again be as a research fellow for a short time period or in a more formal educational capacity, such as an MD or PhD.

3. Review the game plan

Having secured some interval employment, focus can be turned on the unsuccessful application process itself. The worst approach would be to have a 'their problem not mine' attitude and carry on applying exactly as before. You may well be right, maybe it was just bad luck; it is more likely that things can be done next time around to improve your chances of success. So start at the beginning – review your application game plan.

- *Rethink location*
  If relocation is an option, it's definitely time to consider whether this really would be quite as unacceptable as it originally seemed; clearly the more deaneries to which you apply the more chances of success you have.

- *Rethink specialty*
  Your specialty choice also needs to go under the spotlight. It is more than necessary to review whether you have the skills and achievements to make you competitive in this field. Look at the applicants who you know were appointed. How do you differ from them? Are the missing pieces retrievable within

a reasonable time-frame? It is also worth thinking laterally about other similar specialties that you could apply to, or even completely unrelated ones. Remember, there is no restriction on the number of applications you make, so you could still pursue 'the dream' while putting in place a few safety nets. Consider your choices carefully though; the rest of your career is a very long time to spend doing something you hate.

- *Find and use a mentor*
  Locate a senior specialist in your field of interest and obtain an independent opinion of your likelihood of successful appointment in their field. Be prepared to hear some unpleasant truths, but in the long run this crucial check could save you wasting time in search of a dream that is far removed from reality. Alternatively, being given the green light can act as a valuable confidence boost.

4. Re-applying: perfecting that form

So having established your strategy, it's now time to consider the application form at length. For individuals who were not even shortlisted, the problem probably lies back with the application form itself. It is very difficult to find insight into the problems after having spent so long on the form so try the following formula.

- *Make sure that you're ticking all the boxes*
  Start by checking the basic details of your form against the eligibility criteria for the posts you were applying for – do you have all the essential criteria and experience required? Have you made this clear enough in the way you've filled out the form? Have you made any errors in terms of data entry? It happens more often than you'd think!

- *Maximize achievement point scoring*
  Shortlisting scores and the interview cut-off points can be obtained through personal contact with deaneries. You may find it helpful to know just how close to the mark you were. Try to identify where you could have gained those extra crucial points, and set about addressing your identified areas of weakness. Not enough audit? Easily corrected – do one, even something simple is fine as long as you can write or talk about it. Lacking publications? Fine – find yourself a case report to write, submit

a comment or letter on an article or study of interest to you, or try to get involved with any research going on in your hospital and get this acknowledged on any emerging published work. Did insufficient experience let you down? Again, that's not an insurmountable issue; use this interval between training jobs to build your experience in your desired specialty.

5. Phase two: interviews

- *Postmortems are the way forward*
  If interviews were your stumbling block in the previous round, try to work out why. Note down the questions you were asked, along with your answers (if memory allows!) and ask colleagues, both peers and seniors, how they would have answered them. Did you misunderstand what was being asked? Were your answers not structured enough to get your points across clearly? It should quickly become apparent what let you down – now address it!

- *Use the experience of others*
  Interviews run to a very similar format all over the country, and by talking to others you will gain awareness of different themes, scenarios and methods of questioning or practical skills assessments used. This is particularly important at senior levels, where some in-depth specialty knowledge can be expected. Direct your efforts towards areas that come up repeatedly rather than an obscure part of the specialty, and build on the experience of others – this means you are less likely to repeat their mistakes.

- *Practise, practise, practise*
  There really can be no substitute. However you can manage it the more practise you have at answering questions, the more clear, coherent and confident you will come across on the day. Only by speaking out loud will you become aware of your habit of saying 'errrm ...' at the beginning and end of each sentence; seemingly innocuous habits could be really irritating to an observer, and once uncovered must be eradicated!

On the whole you get out what you put in. By ensuring you're fully eligible, choosing specialties and deaneries sensibly, putting in a watertight application and following that up with a solid interview performance, you really will have maximized your chances. With a bit of luck on your side, you'll find you're away and running ... congratulations ... and good luck for the rest of your career!

Do:

- Stay focused

- Reconsider everything

- Apply as much effort as you can expend

- Involve others

Don't:

- **Take things personally**

- **Give up immediately**

- **Be resistant to change**

- **Try to go it alone**

Alternatives for your future

Especially if this is not the first unsuccessful application, or the whole process and career have failed to live up to your aspirations and expectations, you may want to consider alternative options. Barriers to leaving will include financial constraints, and a personal desire not to 'waste' the years spent at university.

Using and developing your skills and experience and common alternatives to the NHS

A medical degree is a valuable commodity. It is proof of hard work and educational achievement; over and above this, it is evidence of the 'non-clinical' transferable skills:

- Teamwork and management
- Communication skills
- Decision making and leadership
- Coping under pressure and prioritization.

All of these are demanded by modern business and a range of employers. The global health-care industry is thriving, and within the NHS there is an increasing focus on training doctors for a management role. In the private sector, consultancy firms now hold recruitment events to specifically target doctors. It should also not be forgotten that the NHS is not the only place to practise medicine.

Pharmaceutical medicine

Pharmaceutical medicine was recognized as a specialty in its own right in 2002. There is significant crossover with research or academic medicine, and a doctor must be able to demonstrate 4 years' experience in appropriate specialties to be eligible for ST in pharmaceutical medicine (http://www.fpm.org.uk).

Military medicine

The armed forces require doctors specializing in general practice and a range of hospital specialties. As well as a reasonable level of physical fitness, aspiring military doctors must demonstrate leadership ability and aptitude for work under pressure. The level of competition within certain specialties remains high, and minimum time commitments apply, of 4 years and upwards. Careers can be in the Army, Royal Navy or the Royal Air Force (http://www.armyjobs.mod.uk).

Medicolegal work

Opportunities for working in the medicolegal sphere range from work as an expert witness, to training and practising as a barrister. Expert witnesses are doctors with significant clinical and/or research experience, who may provide opinions for the court in addition to their clinical workload. In order to work as a solicitor or barrister, a doctor will require further professional qualifications, and competitive entry to a training contract, or 'pupilage' (http://www.mps.org.uk, http://www.the-mdu.com, http://www.lawsociety.org.uk).

Working overseas and out of programme experience (OOPE)

Working in a developing country, through organizations such as Voluntary Service Overseas (http://www.vso.org.uk) and Médecins Sans Frontières (http://www.msf.org.uk) may be incorporated into ST as 'out of programme experience'. The MMC *Gold Guide* sets out the deaneries' expectations and requirements in this regard. It is unusual for doctors to do this for a prolonged period of time, as often you may receive little or no pay.

Alternatively, you may consider working abroad for the longer term. The main destination for UK graduates is currently Australia or New Zealand. Applicants wishing to stay for the longer term should be aware that they may be required to pass various examinations, including the Australian Medical Council exams, and those for the relevant postgraduate college.

Preparing in advance to leave

Working as a junior doctor offers many opportunities to become involved in non-clinical activities. These range from roles within the doctors' mess, or hospital representative committees, through to national roles within the British Medical Association (BMA). NHS Foundation Trusts have specific roles in staff governorship, for which junior doctors are eligible to apply such as a 'local negotiating committee'. Similarly, participation in clinical research may offer valuable experience relevant to pharmaceutical medicine; writing articles for journals may pave the way to a career in medical journalism.

Many non-clinical roles rely on a certain degree of clinical experience. It may be worth obtaining a further qualification, for example, a graduate diploma in law (GDL), or management degree (e.g. MBA). These can be completed part-time, leaving the option of full- or part-time clinical work. Enrolling on a full-time course is also an option for some people. The British Association of Medical Managers (BAMM) (http://www.bamm.co.uk) offers support for doctors considering a career in medical management, and similar programmes are offered by private corporate employers. These may be preferable to 'going it alone' in higher education.

Away from the hospital, you may be able to secure work experience and networking opportunities.

Competing for jobs

Doctors have traditionally competed for jobs based on evidence of experience, and progression to postgraduate qualifications. When applying for a position outside of clinical medicine, these academic achievements may be of lesser importance. Your CV should focus more on the skills and experience you could bring to the role, rather than simply listing your qualifications. Think about your everyday role; emphasize those skills that are important for the new career. Examples include decision making, communication, teamwork and leadership, and the ability to prioritize and function under pressure. Try to demonstrate how your skills are transferable to a new role, and be prepared to sell yourself.

Interview processes vary between organizations; however, a series of interviews or more lengthy attendance at an assessment centre could be expected. You should use the interview process itself to help decide whether you will 'fit in' to the organization.

References will usually be sought as part of the interview process. This is a potential minefield, since commitment to a specific medical career is seen as a prerequisite to the award of a training number. If possible, discuss the issues with your potential employer: they may be content to consult referees only once a provisional job offer is made. Alternatively, you may be able to use referees outside your current specialty or hospital.

Conclusion

A career in medicine incorporates an incredibly diverse range of subspecialties, each offering different challenges, and appealing to different people with different skill sets. Leaving clinical medicine is not a decision to be taken lightly, but equally, should not be discounted entirely. If you do leave, and subsequently wish to return, this will usually require a great deal of effort.

- Try to think about what motivates you – is it the clinical contact, the academic aspects, or the high pressure 'adrenaline' situations? Is it more the financial gain?

- If you enjoy being a doctor, look at non-traditional medical specialties (e.g. public health, legal medicine, advisory roles to industry, or pharmaceutical medicine), before looking outside medicine entirely.

- Develop your transferable skills; get involved in the doctors' mess, local negotiating committee or BMA junior doctors' committee.

- Research the role thoroughly. If possible, speak to other doctors who have made the move.

- Restructure your CV to focus on skills, not simply qualifications. How is your experience relevant to the role you want?

- If you do decide to leave the NHS, try to do so on good terms. You may well end up working within health-care in a different capacity, or indeed want to return to medicine at some point in the future.

Index

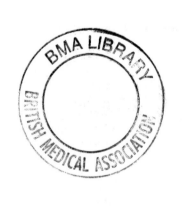